Behind the Mask

of

Parkinson's Disease

LAVONNE UPTON

Personal Conversations with Parkinson's
Patients and Their Loved Ones

THE GIFT: A POEM

by Lavonne Upton

SPOUSE	PARKINSON'S PATIENT
Look at me	*I am. I stare.*
Be still	*I can't. I shake.*
Smile	*I think I am.*
Talk to me	*You can't hear me.*
Reason with me	*Wait for my thoughts.*
Walk with me	*I stumble.*
Hurry up	*I fall.*
Eat with me	*I choke.*
Sleep with me	*I can't get into bed.*
Go out with me	*I can't get dressed.*
Wait here for me	*I forget where I am.*
You make me so angry	*...but I brought you flowers.*

BEHIND THE MASK

OF

PARKINSON'S DISEASE

INTRODUCTION

Encouraged by Harriett Marenas, a member of the Rochester Parkinson's Disease Support Group, Lavonne Upton has written the stories of many of the group's Parkinson's patients and their caregivers. Not only is Lavonne a writer, but she has Parkinson's disease herself. Having two brothers with Parkinson's, one of whom died from complications of the disease, further motivated her.

Nancy Knitter, Harry Knitter (deceased), Pat Yarnold, and Merle Smith founded the Rochester Parkinson's Disease Support Group in 2006, with the help of the Michigan Parkinson Foundation.

The purpose of sharing the stories of the Parkinson's families, and how they cope on a day-to-day basis, is to help others and let them know that they are not alone. Every person represented in this book has graciously given of themselves with honesty, openness, and humor.

Lavonne Upton has done the interviewing, compiling, editing, and writing which has culminated in this publication.

PREFACE

Over the past several months, I met with more than fifty people consisting of individuals, couples, and relatives to interview them about their experiences living with Parkinson's disease. We met at their homes or at a restaurant. Sometimes we met at a coffee shop, and I was so engrossed in their story, I hardly noticed the smoothie machine loudly whirring in the background.

The interviews always lasted longer than planned. Instead of 1 1/2 hours, they effortlessly lasted from 2 1/2 to 3 hours. Even then, most people continued to sit there, not really in a hurry to leave. Some mentioned that it was the first time anyone had heard their entire story.

To make writing this book more manageable, I thoughtfully constructed questions in advance and, with computer in hand, captured a record of our conversations. The intent was to capture as complete a picture as possible of what the Parkinson's patient and caregiver experience regarding their disease, both physically and emotionally.

The Parkinson's patient and their caregiver were asked to answer as if they were speaking in first person. I compiled a notebook about four inches thick of wonderful information from these generously open people.

Since the interviews are to remain anonymous, pronouns are used to identify the person speaking without using their proper name. To be true to the nature or style of the interview, I presented stories in the manner in which the interview was conducted. Some interviews were combined because the spouse was present and interjected their thoughts. Others were separated because the spouse did not want to talk in front of the patient. In several cases, some spouses gave most of the interview as the Parkinson's patient wandered off.

When sequestered away to edit, the hardest part was culling the answers to the carefully worded questionnaire, lest the slightest word edited out be the very tidbit that could be helpful to someone.

The chapters are arranged from the most recently diagnosed person to the person diagnosed the longest. However, this order does not represent how long the person has exhibited symptoms. Please work your way to the back where I also have stories by surviving spouses and, in one case, a surviving daughter.

The title, *Behind the Mask of Parkinson's Disease,* was chosen because of the odd and somewhat vacant look on the face of most Parkinson's patients. This expressionless facade belies the personality of the real person you will discover as you look beyond their appearance.

Behind the mask of these Parkinson's patients I see bright, witty, and humorous persons. They demonstrate an enormous amount of perseverance, courage, wisdom, and willingness to participate in this project.

It has been my privilege to have them share with me their everyday struggles and victories in living with, suffering with, and surviving with, the aggravating, though maybe not life-threatening, incurable, and degenerative disease.

From these conversations, you will be able to go into their homes and see how they cope after they leave the doctor's office.

After reading these stories, other patients, doctors, families, caregivers, and the population at large will certainly better understand what it feels like to live with the debilitating effects of this degenerative disease.

THE MASK

The following are descriptive words or expressions used by the Parkinson's patients themselves, or their loved ones, to describe their facial appearance.

Expressionless face

Having a dour look

No emotions in the face

Stone-face

Downward curve to the mouth

Masking

Face not animated

Looking mad

Looking placid on the outside

Looking drawn

Blank facial expression

Looking tired

Look of not enjoying oneself

Staring blankly

A different look to the face

Unblinking

Drooping in the face

Unhappy looking

Looking like a grouch

Not smiling

Off in another world

Disinterested

CONTENTS

MY STORY

By Lavonne Upton

DIAGNOSED: 4 Days
AGE: 75

I had waited anxiously for months to get a diagnosis. Monday, August 1, finally came. For my 1:40 p.m. appointment, I was early. I had never been to his office before, and I had to drive twenty-five miles to get there. I didn't want anything to interfere with this long-awaited appointment with the neurologist who specialized in movement disorders. It took him only minutes. "You have Parkinson's," he said. As I sat in front of him, he could tell right away the type of tremors I had from my shaking hand on my knee. He noticed a little "masking" that was already occurring in my face. He continued to do a series of tests. I asked, upon leaving, "Would you indulge me a minute longer so I can write down my symptoms?" He said, "They are too numerous for you to write down. You have over fifty symptoms." I said, "Well, my daughter told me I under-react to things." He said, "You have by about five years."

I noticed the tremors in my right hand about five years ago. My, then, primary doctor said they were just benign tremors that come with age and heredity. I believed him. My brother had them. My girlfriend, the same age as I, also had them, and her doctor told her the same thing. She had a brother with them, too. I didn't give any credence to the fact that my brother in California was told he had Parkinson's syndrome several years ago. I thought he was being a little over-reactive to get sympathy. Now five years later, I have to eat crow and realize my pooh-poohing his symptoms have come back to bite me.

My symptoms became more prevalent or noticeable after I moved in February from my large home into a

1

small apartment in a nearby community. Not only does my hand shake, other parts of my body shake, including my whole arm, my shoulder, and when I'm lying down, my side, and my back. My leg shakes, sometimes violently, especially when I feel stressed.

My voice has been gravelly for several years. The same primary doctor said it was from GERD, called GERD laryngitis. It hasn't gotten better; it's gotten worse. A soft or gravelly voice is a common symptom of Parkinson's.

My tremors accelerated in severity. Other strange-occurring things continued to get my attention. I've been saying, for the last year, "Something is not right." I can no longer brush my teeth with my right hand. Months ago, I would try to brush my teeth and think, "This feels funny." It feels like my arm had been asleep and started to wake up but didn't fully wake up. I could not put enough pressure on my hand to brush. I finally switched hands and now brush with my left hand.

About a year ago, it began to feel very unpleasant to bear down to write. I couldn't put much pressure on my hand, and as I wrote, the letters got smaller and smaller, and the pressure weaker and weaker. The words became illegible. I try to avoid making notes, or grocery lists, or to-do lists. At the bank, I have the bank teller fill out my deposit slip. The unpleasant feeling is like when your foot's asleep and you try to stand up and walk but have no strength.

My legs feel heavy. I walk at least three times a day with my dog. I noticed my footprints in the snow last winter, and there was about a ten-inch drag from my right foot after each step. I feel heavy from the hips down, weak-kneed and stiff, as if I can't lift my legs to walk without shuffling. My calves and my legs feel lazy from the hips down. I can't push my right foot into a shoe. There's no strength behind it.

I stumble. I fell several times when in my storage area, looking through my belongings, and in my garage when trying to sort out boxes from my move. I fell off a chair on Easter Sunday at a family gathering.

My tremors cause me to feel jittery and I tense up, trying to "hold on" tight to something to control them. Sometimes I shake all day. I feel like my teeth almost chatter. The phone shakes severely when I hold it to my ear to talk.

I worry that, when I drive, my foot or leg won't respond on the pedals fast enough when necessary.

My legs tremble when I'm standing at the bathroom mirror putting on face creams.

I can't put on or take off a jacket easily.

My right arm clings to my side, instead of swinging normally and freely like my left arm does.

My shoulders become extremely achy and tired-feeling, which can only be relieved by lying down.

I choke easily and frequently on food, and often on my own saliva.

It is becoming a social problem, as I hate to eat out. I drop salad off my fork. I haven't been able to eat soup for years. I long ago learned to hold my glass in my left hand.

It is becoming a problem working, which I do one day a week for a financial advisor. I can't write easily, my writing becomes smaller and smaller, and I have no pressure behind it. The page won't duplicate dark enough on the copy machine. I get tired easily. I limit my workday to three hours, resting in between. I feel edgy and restless around people because of the tremors going on in my body, though maybe unseen to others.

I lost a younger brother to Parkinson's 12 years ago. As I mentioned, I have an older brother living with it in California. Combining that information with the above symptoms, I began to put the pieces together. However, before the neurologist's diagnosis, others didn't take me seriously. I still put on my makeup and dressed up, and they would say, "You look good," like nothing's wrong. It seems they chalked my symptoms up to aging, or complaining.

I had already consulted another neurologist back in April. I had waited anxiously for two months to get in to see her. I had taken my daughter with me. After all my anxiety waiting for this day, the doctor blew me off within minutes, saying I had benign tremors because I was too old to have Parkinson's, which shows up in the 50s. That is such a gross mistake. Parkinson's can still show up in your 60s, 70s, 80s and 90s. I asked her to explain my symptoms; she didn't. I showed her my handwriting. She said, "It doesn't look that bad to me." I was taking medication for benign tremors – the wrong medication for my problem. She tripled the dose. Getting the wrong doctor and a wrong diagnosis has been a frustrating, but common, problem among Parkinson's disease patients.

Fortunately, I volunteer at the senior center with a woman whose husband had Parkinson's. She was his caretaker for ten years before his death and was very familiar with Parkinson's and its symptoms. She was furious about the first neurologist's casual assessment. She gave me the number of the Michigan Parkinson Foundation. I called there and they encouraged me to see a neurologist with an extended education as a movement specialist. I chose a doctor from a list given me. He, as anyone else familiar with Parkinson's, was angry at the first neurologist's flippancy and inability to see the obvious. He could see immediately that "at-rest" tremors, such as mine, are only associated with Parkinson's. He said, "There is no other explanation for them."

After his diagnosis Monday, I attended a Parkinson's disease support group on Wednesday night at the nearby hospital. I saw people in all stages of Parkinson's. It was obvious that the diagnosis for me was accurate. I could identify with most everyone there.

A disturbing piece of information I found out is that Parkinson's is not only a movement disorder, as your brain won't tell your muscles how to move, but also a neurological and psychiatric disorder, as it also affects behavior, such as depression, hallucinations, and almost always leads to dementia.

I was a fashion and photographic model over the years from age 17. In fact, my last gig was at age 62 as a centerfold for *Sunset Magazine* in a polka dot bathing suit on an inner tube in the Pacific Ocean in Del Mar, California, for the Chamber of Commerce of San Diego.

The once tall stature of a fashion model, carrying the latest designs in fashion, is slowly turning into a stooped woman, an inevitable prognosis for a Parkinson's victim; the once freeze framed face, often photographed, slowly turning into a frozen, mask-like one, due to a degenerative, incurable disease.

[Update, three weeks later]

Since the diagnosis three weeks ago, I started medication. I'm only taking a beginning dose. I feel emotionally and mentally good. I still tremor quite a bit and sometimes I feel edgy. I feel a little dizzy sometimes, but not bad. My walking is better. I don't seem to be as wobbly. My legs feel kind of stiff at times, but I don't worry about falling so much, though I seem to veer often. My right side is affected. I think my face is taking on a little masking. I feel like I look different when I look in the mirror. In a way, it doesn't seem like a bad thing; my face just looks more relaxed to me. It still feels unpleasant to write. My arm feels rigid, but I force myself to write three journal pages every morning.

I live alone. I started worrying about the future and my decline – how fast would it be? How incapacitated would I become? How helpless would I be? Would I be able to live alone and take care of myself? Would I be able to drive? I talked to my daughter, who lives out of state. She said, "Mom, you can always come live with us." While that's very comforting to know, I like my life here, my friends, my church, my groups, and my space.

[Today, two years later]

There are still a lot of unpleasant symptoms, and the tremors are still extremely annoying, but it has only hampered my lifestyle a little. I get restless when I go out socially for any length of time because I'm trembling and jittery, or because I get tired. None of this is enough to stop me except when extremely fatigued. Then I give myself permission to lie down if I need to. I no longer work.

I get up every morning forgetting I have limitations and thinking I can conquer the world. Even though my legs are very stiff, I know they will feel better once I'm up and moving. Then I start to clean and, after shaking one small rug, I'm exhausted. I'm so glad to know other people with Parkinson's. We can share and understand one another. I still feel afraid sometimes.

STAYING ACTIVE FOR MY GRANDKIDS

AGE: 66
DIAGNOSED: 18 Months
HE: Parkinson's Patient
SHE: Spouse

SHE: He had tremors and was shuffling his feet. We went to our family doctor. The family doctor suspected Parkinson's disease (PD), and he recommended we go to a neurologist to confirm his diagnosis.

HE: When we went to the neurologist, he knew why we were there. He did a series of tests. He would get behind me and push my shoulder, then he had me tapping my feet, and touching my fingertips. He had me walk, and I couldn't walk with one step in front of the other. My handwriting was pretty much gone. It's very small and I write up hill. Sometimes I can interpret it and sometimes I can't.

SHE: He walks with the same side arm and leg moving. When I walk naturally, I walk right leg left arm forward, left leg, right arm forward. I told him to practice being the toy soldier.

HE: The doctor said I could have had the symptoms for four or five years. He put me on something.

SHE: He was a zombie. He couldn't stay awake. He was dysfunctional.

HE: Then he put me on another medication. It's helped; I don't think I have as many tremors. The doctor mentioned I am showing a little bit of masking. My wife says I seem to be staring ahead occasionally.

SHE: The doctor said to my husband, "Even though you may be happy, the person next to you may not think you are because your face doesn't show emotions." He has a masked look and is rigid when he tries to get up and down, and move.

HE: It's hard to get up. When I get up out of a chair, I try to get myself to stand up straight, but my normal posture is kind of bent from the waist. I start shuffling slowly, but after several steps, my posture becomes more erect, and I can walk faster and more normal. I'm self-conscious of being stooped. She is always telling me, "Straighten up your shoulders. Pick up your feet." I fell two or three times before I was diagnosed. Since then, I've come close, but I haven't fallen at all.

I have tremors on both sides, but more on the right. My hand shakes badly when I try to eat and when I'm trying to trim my mustache.

SHE: When he was trying to eat, it looked like he was wondering how he would get the food up to his mouth. Now he bends down to eat.

HE: I'm conscious of not being able to eat with my right hand too well. I may end up training myself to use my left hand, because it's steadier.

SHE: When someone else is around...

HE: ...even the kids, I hate sitting there shaking. At church, too, instead of sitting at a table with others, I go in the kitchen and eat by myself.

I have more saliva in my mouth than I ever had before. I also notice I stutter a little bit. My wife notices it, but no one else does. I get leg cramps occasionally, and after a long walk, my legs feel really tight; same thing with my shoulders.

SHE: As soon as we start walking, he says, "My shoulders are killing me."

HE: My lower back gets really tight when I get up from the sitting position, or when we go for a walk sometimes.

SHE: If he tries to pick something off the floor, he just can't do it because of rigidity.

HE: I went to BIG and LOUD therapy so that my voice wouldn't fade so fast; it was continuing to get softer and softer. I knew that soon I wouldn't be able to hold a conversation. I try not to let it handicap me now. I try to speak louder, but when we drive to my daughter's, which is 1 1/2 hours away, my wife accuses me of not talking to her.

I'm concerned about my driving, because she tells me I'm speeding or I'm going too slow, and I'm swerving from one lane to another. The doctor doesn't want me to drive long distances.

SHE: Sometimes he's crawling, and sometimes he's speeding. I feel bad, and I try not to say anything unless it's extreme. It seems like he can only concentrate on one thing.

HE: I have glaucoma. My ophthalmologist mentioned something about my eye-blinking right after I went to the neurologist.

SHE: He doesn't blink his eyes as much. He has dry-eye.

HE: Most of the time, my hands are cold now. When I get chilled, my right arm jerks, shaking badly.

SHE: He has shaken all over, big time; it's kind of scary.

HE: Therapy has taught me a technique to get out of bed that I utilize sometimes. I have another situation where I almost pass out from lightheadedness. A book the doctor gave me said it's caused by two factors – a drop in blood pressure and dehydration.

SHE: He's always done his own, but he started coming to me almost every Sunday, asking me to button his shirt. I thought, "Does he want attention or what?"

HE: A headache comes on the left side of my head from front to back, and lasts about 20 seconds. The pain is pretty intense. The neurologist said recent tests on my carotid artery showed nothing, so they said the medicine, which has worked for almost two years, may be causing it. The doctor thinks that increasing one of the meds should help.

SHE: I think his appetite has changed. Other than sweets, he doesn't get excited about eating. He'll say, "Yes, it's OK."

HE: Everything kind of tastes the same. I've lost 45 pounds over three years. I used to say, "Wow, that really smells good," when she was cooking dinner. I don't do that anymore because I can't smell.

Before I got my sleep machine, I had trouble sleeping. I went for the sleep tests and agreed I had very bad sleep apnea.

SHE: The sleep disorder goes along with Parkinson's. We found we're not the only ones that had this weirdness going on. He would act out his dreams; he was usually chasing someone or being chased. He would laugh and sound like another person.

HE: I would go to bed at night, and I'd end up with everything torn off the bed. I'd punch the dresser, and my hand would be bleeding. I injured my heel when I fell out of bed. I'd see things that weren't really there while sleeping, and punch my wife. By cutting the medication in half, I no longer have the problem and smaller dosages still control the involuntary movements I had.

SHE: He has more anxiousness than he did before. I try to keep things written down that he's going to do each day.

HE: I'm a little more timid, a little more anxious. I probably want things to go better than I did before. I can't remember things like I did.

SHE: He seems to have some confusion, but it is real short term. He'll wonder where we are, but then shortly, he's OK.

HE: When the doctor confirmed I had PD, being a pretty emotional person, I shed a couple of tears. At first I thought, "Why me?" But then I thought, "There are some things that Parkinson's can't take away from me: my wife, my God, my children, my grandchildren." I'm going to try to have the best attitude I can, no matter how tough it is, I'm going to be tougher.

We were both born in the south. We met when I was playing baseball on a church team. I've been in sales just about my whole life, as a store manager or outside sales.

SHE: We have two daughters and two grandkids that live nearby. Just like us, they knew that something was not right. The oldest one is a lot like her dad – competitive. She's had him going to the gym with her. She's not going to let Parkinson's get him down. There's probably a little bit of denial with me and the girls, too. Sometimes denial is easier.

HE: Our sons-in-law have been very supportive, also. We have a close family. We have a lot of love.

SHE: I try not to let it affect our lifestyle. It's an inconvenience sometimes because we can't do what we'd like to do.

HE: We still do quite a bit. We're both very active in our church. We walk when we can, and exercise daily at home. I just started a Tai Chi class. We have two couples we go to dinner and the theatre with. I try to keep a good attitude. Some days are pretty good, but it's like something is gnawing at you all the time. My concern is that one day I'll lose my mobility and won't be able to get around on my own, or that one day I will need a full time caregiver. I realize I've got to stay active to keep it at bay as long as I can.

SHE: I want to be there to support him to be the best that he can be.

HE: I don't want the day to come when my wife will have to take me to the bathroom and do all those personal things. I get anxiety about it, even though she's very supportive. If something's not right, she's pretty dynamic about handling things.

SHE: I think he's more emotional now that he has Parkinson's. He was struggling with depression for at least a year before he was diagnosed, and is on a very low dose of medication for it. The Parkinson's support group has been great for both of us; talking to others, you realize you're not alone. All the information they provide has been very helpful.

HE: I would advise others with symptoms to go to the doctor and find out what's going on. Women are more prone to go than men. I had never before been to the doctor as much as I have since I've been diagnosed.

I guess the hardest thing to cope with is the realization it's always there. You get a little period where you feel pretty good. Michael J. Fox said this and it's happened to me – "I have a few good days and then I look at my little finger and it's moving, like saying, 'Hey I'm still here.'"

Friends don't really know where you're coming from. The people in the Parkinson's support group can relate to you more. It's comforting.

I enjoy football more than anything. I used to like to bowl. I'd like to bowl again. I enjoy reading; I've read a lot of motivational and self-help books about business. I'm pretty fortunate that I have several men's groups I meet with regularly, and have male friends that I talk to just about every day. They've been very supportive. We have our church family that we value.

SHE: We have our own space.

HE: She does pretty much what she wants to do. I do pretty much what I want to.

My wife has probably helped me the most, and the kids calling to see how I'm doing. I want to stay active for my grandchildren.

LAUGH AT YOURSELF

AGE: 60
DIAGNOSED: 18 Months
Female Parkinson's Patient

I was diagnosed 18 months ago. The first thing my neurologist told me was that I wasn't blinking as much as normal. The doctor could see the masking in my face, but the everyday person probably couldn't. Myself, I never thought it showed until I saw a picture of me. It was weird because my face just looked blank. My girlfriend's daughter saw the picture of me, too, and asked, "What's the matter with her face?" I can see why it is referred to as a mask.

If I stay calm and take my meds, I'm OK, but during the night, when my meds have worn off, I have tremors and restless leg syndrome really bad. And stress really triggers the tremors.

My stooping has gotten better since I went through the LSVT BIG therapy six months ago. I didn't walk big, and I didn't swing my arms. It's a fantastic program. I don't stoop as much now; my posture's better. The people there are so super nice, calming, and laid back.

I've fallen three times so far because of my shuffling. The meds have helped that. One time I went to turn around, and I didn't turn. I froze. I just waited a second to collect my thoughts, and then I could turn.

I don't notice anything wrong with my voice, as I've always been kind of quiet, but everybody says, "Speak up. I can't hear you."

My movements are really slow right now. I used to be a pretty vibrant person where I'd go, go, go. Now my legs feel like rubber bands most of the time. Five months ago, I thought I could run into the store without a cart. I made it to the back of the store to get an item, but an employee had to help me get back up front. I've always been a big shopper, but now walking is my biggest challenge. Because of my rubbery knees, I feel like I'm going to collapse.

It got to the point, just before I was diagnosed, that I couldn't get in bed. I crawled in like a dog. Then, I couldn't get out. I couldn't sleep. I felt crawly feelings in my arms and legs. Heat really helped me before I started on medication. The medication has been a godsend. I also wear a patch, which helps my meds be more effective for my particular problems. I change it every 24 hours.

Most of the time I do pretty well, but sometimes, if I get down on the floor, I have a hard time getting up. I have a Styrofoam™ roll suggested by the LSVT BIG therapy to be used to help straighten out my spine. I can't get off it. The other day I couldn't get off the couch. I couldn't get my legs around. So I just fell on the floor.

I had a frozen shoulder before I went to therapy. It's been bothering me again the last couples of weeks. My whole right side was stiffening up and I couldn't use it. I don't swing my right arm and my right hand is weak.

I had to buy an electric toothbrush because I don't have the strength to brush hard enough. I've pretty much become left handed. The physical therapist kept telling me to use my right hand. My neurologist told me that PD will eventually affect both sides.

My appetite is good as ever. Love the sweets.

I noticed I didn't have a sense of smell for a couple of years before my diagnosis. It happened so slowly, I didn't really pay attention to it until I couldn't even smell a skunk. That's when I thought it was really weird.

I got so I couldn't order steak in a restaurant because my husband would have to cut it for me. I went out to lunch with my girlfriend last week, and I couldn't cut my salad.

People at work commented to me how tired I looked and asked me, "Is your back hurting you?" I was starting to slouch over. Eighteen months ago, my stepdaughter graduated from high school and we had an Open House with over 100 people. Probably 90 people commented to me or my daughter about how I was. A couple of friends commented my hands were shaking. I went to my primary doctor and told him about my concerns. He sent me to a neurologist. I was in denial, I guess, because the symptoms were so weird – like I couldn't get into bed. And once I got in to bed, I couldn't roll over. I felt like I was sticking like Velcro®. He wasn't a movement disorder specialist and I wasn't happy with him, so a year later, I went to a movement specialist. She switched my meds a little bit, and she added a patch a month ago.

I have very vivid dreams every night from the time I go to sleep until I wake up; weird, off-the-wall dreams. I've dreamed about every person I've ever known in my life, people I haven't seen in 30 years. I'd wake up and say, "Where did that come from?"

My fatigue level varies from day to day. I get drowsy about 20 minutes after medication. I don't sleep very well at night. I'm kind of restless.

I was angry mad when I left the doctor's office. I was in kind of a state of shock. I thought I'd cry, but I didn't. I called my daughter when I got home. She said, "Come on mother, what's the deal?" When I told her, she started crying. I said, "Now you know why I've been the way I have." She said, "Don't worry. We'll get through it."

We did passports at work. I couldn't write the information off their drivers' license into the little box. My boss said, "Why can't you write?" If I took information over the phone, I wasn't able to decipher what I had written. I was stumbling around the back room. It was a disaster. My husband finally said, "Just give up your job."

My husband has ADHD, and is a very, very hyper, workaholic. He's very caring but off in his own world most of the time. He freaked out when I told him. He's in total denial and won't talk about it. He'll change the subject and just say, "My wife is sick."

I was very depressed at first, but then I thought, "I'll just do as much as I can." It bothers me, though, that I can't spend as much time with my grandkids. I'm too fatigued and my legs get too funky, real rubbery, when I drive that far – four hours – to see them; the restless leg kicks in. Sometimes I think my restless leg is worse than my PD. I have it every night. The medication, I have six all together, helps a little bit, but it's trial and error. I would advise others with symptoms to not ignore them. The sooner you get on medication, the better.

I'm afraid I might have to start using a motorized cart at the store. I was told I should be using a cane. I'm not ready to admit I need that yet. I'd rather hold on to a grocery cart. I just don't want to be in a wheelchair.

The girlfriends and I still meet once a month for dinner. My husband and I go out every Saturday night for dinner to a nice restaurant; otherwise we don't have much of a social life.

My husband's daughter came over with her four month old baby. It was disturbing to me that I couldn't get out of the chair and walk around with her for fear of falling.

I have my good days and my bad days. Bad days I'm fatigued and depressed. I can't do the things I used to. I can't keep up. Sometimes I'm a little scared about my situation, but I've had a pretty good run so far. I just think my memory isn't as sharp as it used to be.

To cope, I go get my hair done. I get my nails done, and I use the gift certificates my husband gives me for massages. I started going to family counseling about two weeks ago called "Talk Therapy." My neurologist suggested it. I was bummed that I hadn't gone sooner to the Parkinson's support group, too. I walked in one night and I couldn't tell anyone had PD; they looked like normal people. I was happy about that.

I love bird watching. I have lots of bird feeders outside my bay window. I love to feed the squirrels. I have a pet squirrel that knocks on my window every day. I love going to the baseball games. I watch all sports on TV – basketball, baseball, football, and hockey. I like to sew. I haven't done much lately; in the past, I made all my daughter's clothes.

I'm married, with three children, and seven grandchildren. My husband and I have been together ten years. On Sundays, we ride around and look at property for my husband and his business partner to build on. He is a developer. He works full time as a steam pipefitter. I don't think we're as close as we were. He thinks I've changed; I think he's changed. We've had our ups and downs. He tends to drink more since he's found out about my PD.

The best tip I can think of is "mind over matter." Just try to be positive, because I think symptoms are worse with depression. Try to avoid stress, and be around supportive people. You have to be able to laugh at yourself. My girlfriend and I were laughing about our "diseases." She has Meniere's disease. I said, "You'll be pushing me in a wheelchair, and I'll be telling you where to go."

PATIENCE IS A VIRTUE

AGE: 75
DIAGNOSED: 2 years
HE: Parkinson's Patient
SHE: Spouse

HE: Over the last five years, things have changed about my appearance: my face has less expression, my shoulders hunch, and I shuffle when I walk. My weight has gone down about 25 pounds.

SHE: He never would have gone to the doctor; it was me that made him go.

People may recognize he has Parkinson's disease (PD) by the way he stands, the way his head is forward and his jaw is slack. He stoops, big time. I tell him to straighten up. "OK, tits out," I say. With the masking, his face takes on a disinterested appearance. He doesn't smile much. He's staring off into space half the time. His voice is so low and quiet, I'm always asking, "What did you say?" I used to yell at him to get involved in the conversation, but he withdrew right into himself. He doesn't talk to anyone anymore; he just doesn't get involved, socially.

HE: If I have to talk very loud, I won't do it. I have never been an outgoing type of person. Now I have to force myself, and after I start talking, people can't hear me anyway, unless I yell. I find it's annoying to me and it's annoying to others. I'll say, "good morning," and then I won't talk anymore.

SHE: He worked for Kmart and supervised the transporting and moving of products – getting stuff from warehouses into stores. He didn't plan on early retirement, but he was retired when the company down-sized. He started a little handyman business, refinishing decks and doing landscaping.

HE: I could do anything and everything as a handyman and loved it.

SHE: I worked at the church. Many people, especially widows, came in wanting referrals for handymen. That's how his handyman business started.

HE: I did that for 13 years – up until two years ago.

SHE: One customer finally said, "You can't do that anymore." I thought, "He's just getting older," but now I look back and realize he had PD then."

HE: But I can do a lot of things yet. The only thing is, I put myself at risk. Lifting becomes harder and harder.

SHE: He has a frozen shoulder, and he probably started shuffling about four or five years ago. I'd nag him all the time, saying, "Pick up your feet."

HE: We have this internist I had been going to for 20 years. He would routinely check my blood pressure and say, "You're healthy." One visit, he noticed something and said, "You've got Paget's disease." That's when the leg's bow out. Eventually he recommended I see a neurologist.

SHE: The neurologist diagnosed PD by watching my husband walk, by testing his strength, by his memory, and then put him on medication and told him to come back in a month to see if the shuffling and the drooling was improved.

I called up his brothers and sisters. They said, "We knew something was wrong but we didn't know what." They were glad to have a name for it.

He's been on the medication for two years – ever since he was diagnosed. He started having hallucinations last summer, so we cut back on the dosage. My daughter lives in Boston. He thought she was in the kitchen. Another time, he called the police and told them someone was in the house. I said to him, "You can't be calling the police; the police will get tired of coming and you'll have to go into assisted living."

HE: Yeah, it frightened me. The last time, I heard these people in the house and they were going to steal our TV's. When I looked out, I saw two men carrying them into their car. She said, "You're crazy." I started to go down there to stop them. She said, "There's no one there." If I had a gun I probably would have shot at someone. That's when I called the doctor and said, "Help." He cut back the dosage. I still get hallucinations a little, but not very bad. We were on vacation three or four weeks ago and I thought the dog was there on a chair, so I started walking toward her, and she just vanished.

SHE: He has fallen a couple of times. One time he fell when he went out onto the porch, and he fell in the basement, off a step stool.

HE: I thought, "Oh, a little step stool can't hurt me." I fell backward and thought I broke my pelvis. I could have been badly hurt or dead. It was about ten minutes before I could get up. She wasn't home.

It's tough getting in and out of cars. My writing got worse and worse.

SHE: He hardly writes anything anymore.

HE: I still golf.

SHE: We bowled for 40 years but it got to be too hard on him. He couldn't handle the weight of the ball. He can hardly carry anything down to the basement anymore. He's got to hold on.

HE: It's changed my life. I can't do the windows. I'd fall off the ladder. Virtually, I do nothing. Well, I do the dishwasher, but it's very easy to drop the plates. I like to read books.

SHE: He doesn't read much anymore. When he had that little handyman business, it kept him busy sometimes six days a week.

HE: My wife is a super-duper driver. At night, I don't drive anywhere anymore – even two blocks. She does it all. That's really changed my life.

SHE: One thing he does to unwind: he likes to watch the History Channel on television. The other thing he does when the weather is good is go out on the patio and take a nap with the dog sleeping close by. Sometimes he doesn't think of things to do himself.

HE: I see more and more about Parkinson's on TV. The top advice I'd give to others is to get a specialist. I want to go to a person whose patients are 100 percent Parkinson's patients.

The one thing that affects me is I forget my name sometimes, and my age. My memory was one of my biggest problems long before PD was officially diagnosed. As far as tremors, I don't have any tremors.

SHE: He has trouble getting in and out of bed. He can't seem to get his feet up and under the covers. It takes forever.

HE: When I get out of bed in the morning, I can't get up immediately. I have to get up slowly because I could fall. If my wife wasn't around, I'd definitely need an aid to help me out of bed.

My emotions are on a pretty even keel. My life is kind of great; I've got the greatest person in the world – my wife. And what else can I do? I have problems with buttons. If it wasn't for her, I'd go around naked. It takes me forever to get an undershirt on. I started calling that shirt every name in the book.

SHE: It's hard in the winter; he gets his coat on but his collar is way down in the middle of his back.

HE: My wife doesn't work, so she's my 100% caretaker. I don't worry about it. She takes care of everything. I've got a dog here and it talks to me. I'm totally bored. I feel healthy. I've got a few minor things with PD, but I think I can do everything I did before.

SHE: No, he can't.

HE: My life changed a lot because there's a lot she has to do.

SHE: We used to play cards a lot with all our friends. He has a hard time holding the cards now. We were great pinochle players. Now he forgets what's played and he's lost his competitive spirit. He doesn't seem to accept or recognize his limitations.

HE: At our age, we should know that we're going to have problems. Some are PD. Some are old age.

SHE: In a way, PD is kind of a downer. We've taken a lot of fabulous trips in the past, and he's just not able to handle the suitcases and all that goes along with it anymore. We don't want to go on a trip and have him sleep the whole time on a bus. He poops out easily.

I chum around with ten women, and we go on an annual trip up north to see a dinner show put on by *Young Americans*, young people between the ages of 18-28. I'm involved in church and I take care of my first cousin, age 93, who lives in assisted living. I do all her doctor's appointments and medications. I worked 17 years in Christian service, at a church, and I have been retired for seven years.

The hardest thing to cope with about the disease and his condition is our social life, although I'm pretty good at calling people. We've got some wonderful friends. I'll have them for dinner, or we'll go to a show. They've always called me the "group leader."

I'm trying to develop patience, instead of impatiently saying, "I'm saying it once. Do it. Get it done and over with."

There's a great group of people in our PD support group. The group is as helpful to the caregiver as it is to the patient. My advice would echo what they keep emphasizing: "Keep moving, keep exercising, and keep yourself going."

HUMOR MAKES PEOPLE HAPPY

AGE: 66
DIAGNOSED: 3 years
Male Parkinson's Patient

People I have known for years ask, "What's wrong?" They can't understand what I'm saying, and they ask me to say it again. I used to be outgoing and gregarious and speak publicly without a microphone. Now, I mumble quietly, especially when I'm tired, and my wife often asks, "What did you say?"

I took the LSVT therapy – LOUD. They taught me how to slow down and enunciate my words so they're clear and succinct. To me, my voice seems a normal volume, but it's soft. I would advise others to take the BIG and LOUD courses. In the physical therapy side of it, they showed me how to take larger steps so I can concentrate on walking, which to me seems exaggerated but looks normal. When I shuffle, I remember to try to control my gait, and I try to think like we did in the military – left, right, left, right.

Articles I read tell me some people have a mask, which means their face is less animated. I don't smile as much, and I sometimes have a dour look. I have a downward curve to my mouth.

My wife tells me I am stooping. I have to think about how my balance is, and how my posture is. When I'm speaking, I can only think about speaking. I can't balance all the plates any more. I find I have to concentrate on the topic at hand, and deal with the other issues the best I can. My brain has to think about walking, talking, drooling, and my facial expressions; things that I would never have given thought to before. Multi-tasking is now more difficult with the disease.

My drooling is controlled by keeping my posture vertical, so I'm not stooping, and my head is horizontal.

My first indication that something was going on was about three years ago when my keyboard skills began going away. In the office using the computer, my left side was making mistakes like crazy. If I typed a word, I might get stuck on an "a" and there might be 20 a's in a row. Spell-check was having a meltdown.

My son, who is a paramedic, said he thought maybe I ought to see a neurologist. I went to one where he works. She did the standard testing. When tapping my feet, my left foot was not tapping as well as my right. All of a sudden it wasn't doing it at all. I try to be jovial about it. Considering all other maladies one can run across in life, it seems like a relatively minor thing to deal with. However, at the time, I hadn't read enough about Parkinson's disease (PD) to know what can happen downstream. Some people suggest I make sure if I go to a hospital I go to one that understands PD, and especially PD medications.

I've heard the disease can be attributed to farm chemicals, and automotive chemicals. I own a company that sells and services automotive equipment. Our company builds machines that repair cars, and I'm in and out of automotive shops all the time where they spray chemicals constantly. They spray silicone, penetrating oil, carburetor cleaners, and kerosene based solvents. I don't know what the relationship is between PD and these chemicals. I was also exposed to Agent Orange when I was overseas in Thailand during the Vietnam conflict. Agent Orange was used to kill the surrounding vegetation in the hot and damp jungle. There were drums of it stored around the base. They used to spray the area from spray nozzles on the planes loaded with defoliating chemicals. The chemicals were inside the body of the plane. People were kneeling in it, breathing it in.

I've spent hundreds of hours hunting and doing guy stuff, but I can be emotional, happy and sad, and I'm not sure what causes it. It could be the PD. I get emotional watching a chick flick.

The only balance problem I have is with my check book, at this time.

I was in martial arts for several years and there's a technique of how to fall. You fall hundreds and hundreds of times when you're throwing someone, so you learn how to protect yourself. But it's easier falling on a mat than on concrete.

I get cramping at night. I attribute that to my medication. When trying to get out of bed or turn over, I get bound up in bed clothes. I can't slide. Getting in and out of a car is hard, too. I can't slide over on cloth seats. I have seen a tremor, but it's minimal and only on the left side, but my motion is slow and sluggish. I find that when I get up, I have stiffness from being in one position too long, but once I'm up, I'm OK.

My wife says I have very vivid dreams, but I don't remember them. She said I punched her once in a dream. In my dream, I was actually pushing a tricycle with a child on it. She was the recipient of the push in the form of a punch.

My writing is getting smaller. If I go really slow, I can write somewhat normal, but not like the cursive we learned in grade school. I can button my shirts on the right side fine, but the left side is a struggle.

My first doctor, a neurologist, diagnosed me with Parkinson's. When we found out I had PD, my niece, a Ph.D. in microbiology, got me an appointment with a well-known specialist in the area. Between you, me, and the post, I kind of felt that to him I was only a mild case, and I'm not sure that he put all that much attention onto my case. So I went back to my first neurologist.

I was more curious as to what all was involved with the disease, the prognosis, and what it would be like in the future. I was trying to be proactive. The doctors seem to want you to take small bites of the apple, instead of dropping it all on you up front.

That was roughly three years ago. What was going on then was really minor. I now go to a PD specialist who said often times you can stay at stage one. I thought I might be frozen in time at that stage. In the last six months, however, I seem to be getting an increase in symptoms, such as slowness of movement, drooling, and all the different symptoms that I've mentioned. I believe that the disease is progressing. I'm more aware that I have to designate brain time to control the things I never thought about before, but just did.

I like humor because it makes people happy, in most cases. Humor is just part of what I like to do. I especially enjoy it with my three grandchildren. I can be like a kid again. Some people lose their youth. I don't want to get grumpy, where nothing amuses me or interests me anymore. My mom is 93, still painting within her home. If she can do it, then why can't I?

I have to be careful with safety issues. I have to be careful going down the stairs to my office. I hold the handrail all the time, not just some of the time. I can't go rollerblading any more. I'm no longer motorcycling or pedal biking, although I'm considering buying one of those bicycling/trikes that you have to put a flag on because you sit so low to the ground.

We have two children. Sometimes I think they are too watchful, but they're really not. My wife was going through cancer problems when the boys were teenagers. They stepped up to the plate during that time. They're just good guys. I guess you can consider yourself good parents when others comment about your children's service to family and the community.

I think of all the things I've survived sowing my wild oats; accidents that happened. I'm not fearful of death; it's going to happen one way or the other, sooner or later, so I'm resigned to that fact of life. I've made my peace with God. I guess I don't let it get to me. I don't think about it in the sense that it's overwhelming. I get up every day and put my shoes on and go to work. I haven't gotten so bad that I have to put an "L" or "R" on my shoes. We can't go dancing, though. I feel too robotic trying to do that.

I've never relied on anybody. I've always been one to take care of myself. I go to the support group, though, because I can commiserate with people that are like-afflicted. I'd like to be able to say I'm there to support them, too. I'm fortunate to have a family with a medical background, and one large enough to be a support system to one another.

I came from a large family of seven kids, and I had a sister die when she was two days old. I've been married 39 years. Both our boys live in the area and both are married. The grandchildren are a blast. I have time for them now that I didn't have before because of work.

My wife and I have had only a half dozen arguments in our marriage. She was diagnosed with brain cancer. She's been chemo-ed, radiated, cut on, and has survived over 20 years. By the grace of God, she manages.

The biggest challenge for me is trying to focus on more than one thing at a time.

My best tip is to not be afraid to ask for help if you need it. I was going to put in a light bulb the other day. I should have asked my son, instead of getting on an eight foot ladder. It's a guy thing to want to do it myself.

I don't use chain saws any more. They're very powerful and can buck. I've cut thousands of feet of lumber for firewood or to clear the woods, but, with my slower response time, I can't do it anymore.

A positive thing that's come out of this is having more intimate conversations about me – whereas before it was never about me. I get to talk about me to my family. I've more of a tendency to tell people how I feel. Before, I had a personal face, a family face, a business face. I never really hid anything, but if I had an opinion about something, I might not have mentioned it. Being in sales, too, I was always deferring to the customer. Now I feel like, "Why is my opinion not important?" I guess I allocate time to me. Before that, it was only about my job function to provide for my family.

YOU'RE STILL YOU INSIDE

AGE: 71
DIAGNOSED: 3 years
HE: Parkinson's Patient
SHE: Spouse

HE: At first it was pretty obvious by looking at me that I had Parkinson's disease (PD). I had all the symptoms that go with Parkinson's. I didn't blink my eyes very much. I had the expressionless face. I had no arm motion when I walked, and I shuffled, though not severely. My voice became very faint. It was hard for me, when I'd go to talk, to get words out, my mouth would be so dry. My personal trainer can tell you that I stooped. She can tell you how I've improved.

SHE: What I probably noticed, at first, was he had problems with his arm. He was holding it funny, kind of holding it to the side. He said it hurt a lot, so he went to an orthopedic doctor who gave him some exercises to do. That was about five years prior to diagnosis. Then the next thing I noticed was tremors that he had in his hand. Then the third thing was that his handwriting became small – almost illegible. Another thing was the gradual change in his facial expressions.

HE: Over ten years ago, I noticed a loss of sense of smell. I thought it was old age. I was 58. Other symptoms were my illegible handwriting. And it didn't take much for me to perspire a lot if there was some kind of tension or stress. My eyes were dry. I had loss of strength and loss of grip. The loss of strength was gradual and became a problem. I remember having trouble just pushing my chair back from the table. Trying to get up from my chair was an effort. I was self-conscious when we went out to eat. I could barely handle the knife and fork. I remember once we went to a very fancy restaurant for a dinner meeting and I had to have the cook cut my meat for me. I thought it was a tough steak, but it was my lack of hand strength. And I had this thing where my thumb would fold under and lock up. It was very painful. I had to massage it before I could open it up. It took longer and longer for it to release. I was getting painful cramps in my whole hand. When I slept, I got muscle cramps in my calves. The leg cramps were so bad, they would wake me up. I had loss of flexibility. Now I work out on resistance machines to strengthen my arms and my legs.

SHE: His internist sent him to a neurologist. The neurologist reported back to him that my husband should have a more thorough exam. My husband made a special request to get a copy of the neurologist's summary report. In reading his report, we found out that my husband probably had Parkinson's. His internist didn't pass this information along to my husband. He said, "Well, we're not going to do anything about that until you start shuffling your feet." This made me madder than a hornet. I looked at my husband and said, "We're going back to the neurologist and have it checked further."

HE: I had been diagnosed about 30 years before with bipolar disorder. When my hands started tremoring, I attributed it to the bipolar meds. That was about five years ago, and it was two years until I would be diagnosed with Parkinson's disease. They diagnosed me two years ago at age 68. When they diagnosed me with Parkinson's, along with the bipolar, I went into a pretty severe depression. I found out that's not uncommon.

I went through a period where everything was dark. I would wake up and I was so afraid. Luckily it only lasted a month or so. I was bad, and then I was better. After my PD diagnosis, and during the depression, I lost a lot of weight. I went from 212 to 182 pounds, due to fear and concern, and feelings of doom, with no sense of control. Now I'm back up to my target weight of 193, which I maintain.

The depression was so consuming, my teeth would chatter. The dentist, whom I've gone to for 30 years, made a mouth guard for me. I don't have to worry about teeth chattering anymore. And, as an added benefit, I'm less likely to snore.

SHE: Once we found out he had Parkinson's, I thought, "Well, this is the end of life as we know it." He was moving much slower and was really depressed. He just sat and stared. The severe part lasted at least two to three months. I called his psychiatrist and said, "What do we do here?"

HE: I went to one psychiatrist and two psychologists. We had trouble convincing any of them that Parkinson's triggers depression. After a couple of visits to each psychologist, I said, "This is not going to help me." I had thought I could control the depression by managing my emotions. I blamed myself that I couldn't. Now I know it's chemical and the depression was linked to my Parkinson's. Just recently, a couple of studies show the same mechanism in your brain that creates Parkinson's also often creates depression. In her article, *"Depression is biggest hurdle for Parkinson's patients,"* by Janice Lloyd, USA TODAY [November 28, 2012], she reported that, "A new study shows depression is a bigger challenge than the physical obstacles that patients face."

My son helped me do research on meds. My neurologist said that the bipolar meds I was taking were accentuating the Parkinson's. He suggested an alternative medicine. We finally got the psychiatrist to agree, and that coincided with my recovery from depression.

SHE: We've lived with his having bi-polar disorder. We also saw his step-father suffer from Parkinson's and deteriorate, so we worried about the future and what it would hold. His father was diagnosed with schizophrenia, and his father's sister was committed to a state hospital, but nobody talked about it. Our son is bi-polar, and had severe episodes when in his late 20s. Now he's fine.

HE: My neurologist said Parkinson's disease is not hereditary, but is "familial."

My son's recovery was partly due to medication, and also because he exercises regularly, and does Tai Chi. Once again, exercise increases the blood flow, which somehow flushes and regenerates the brain. First hand, I am an exercise advocate for myself, and my son.

My first neurologist had given me 18 pills to take every day. However, he did order an MRI, CT scan, and an EEG to rule out anything other than PD. Thank God I was told about a movement specialist, whom I changed to. That was the best thing I did. The test for Parkinson's was mostly the movement test in his office, testing my arm flexibility, how I walked, and my stability. He eliminated about half the medications and I only take one now for Parkinson's. But I also take medication for bipolar and depression. I've learned how to manage them to minimize side effects. I don't feel depressed at all anymore.

SHE: Right after his diagnosis with Parkinson's, during his severe depression, he fell getting out of bed. We didn't know what was wrong. He was weak. Our neurologist said, "Take him to emergency." It was a urinary tract infection.

HE: After that experience, I drink water all day long until 9 p.m.

SHE: I hovered too much at the beginning. I worried about leaving him alone. I'd check back in with him often. There were a few falls that scared us. He had fallen in the shower. Now I don't think I treat him any differently. I think I was probably very worried and scared about what the future held. About the time we got his diagnosis, we went on a cruise to Alaska. He seemed very anxious. It was good to get away, but I thought about the Parkinson's all the time. Actually, it was strange because we almost missed a flight connection, and after seeing him be so slow, he ran faster than I've ever seen him, to get to the gate so we wouldn't miss our connection.

HE: When I first started to exercise, I had less than half the capability I have now. Ten minutes and I felt exhausted. Now I walk 40 minutes and I feel fine.

I was very constipated, probably because of the medication and lack of exercise. I've learned to mitigate that problem. I always have fruit at breakfast, and then I drink prune juice when I need to.

To do all the little everyday tasks, such as teeth brushing, I've had to learn new strategies.

SHE: At first I had to button his shirt buttons. The meds have helped, and I no longer have to do that. When he was in depression, I gave him his meds. He's pretty independent now.

HE: I fell four or five times. I'd go to sit on the bed. I'd be in the shower. I'd get up at night. I found it's not good for me to make a rapid movement, like if I try to turn too fast.

There are four factors that help me in my recovery:

- A specialist: A neurologist who is experienced with Parkinson's medical treatment.
- Exercise: With help from someone equipped to work with people with Parkinson's.
- Attitude: The glass is half full instead of half empty. Of course being an engineer, "The glass is twice as big as it needs to be."
- Parkinson's support group: For sharing information and inspiration.

Parkinson's doesn't stop us from doing anything now. During depression, it stopped me from doing everything. I drive now, but during depression, I voluntarily didn't, because I couldn't concentrate enough to drive.

SHE: Once he got on the right dosage of medication, he acted as if he didn't have Parkinson's.

HE: Monthly, we meet with a local chapter of a national organization, where we have dinner, a speaker, and discussion. Once a week I meet for breakfast with my youngest brother, who lives nearby. I go to the local senior center for physical therapy with a personal trainer. Going to that facility is partially social, too. We go on some of their trips and attend some of their musical programs.

SHE: We've lived here in our home for 37 years. As far as coping, I'm pretty stoic. For support, I have coffee every morning, Monday through Friday, with neighbors. I consider them my best friends, and we all encourage one another. I'm a retired nurse, and I volunteer for various community and church programs. I'm able to continue doing what I love doing. I try to exercise regularly. I sew and quilt for family and church.

HE: We attend church a couple of times a month, their monthly breakfast, and their special events. I walk daily in the city park which is only two blocks from our home. We play euchre once a month. I do a lot of crossword puzzles. I study the History of Christianity initiated by watching a PBS television program. Since then, I subscribe to a journal called "Biblical Archeology." I have a stronger faith than I ever did.

SHE: Our social life hasn't suffered. Actually, we're having a whole lot of fun. I think we're closer because we figure out what's important in life, and it's like "Us against PD." We started our bucket list – trips we want to take – and we continue our annual traditional trip up north with our two children, their spouses, and our three grandchildren.

The Parkinson's monthly support group is wonderful. It's been better than I thought it would be. I thought that we'd be depressed to see what the future held, but people are very upbeat. We attend most months. We also go to the monthly breakfast. It is a wonderful group. We've done so much, like the Christmas party, the annual fundraiser gala, and the annual picnic.

HE: I came in there thinking I was doomed. I had been reading about Parkinson's and what was written seemed to be the worst case scenarios. Through the support group, I listened to others share how they kept active. It was inspirational. There are people there that have had Parkinson's 20 years and you can't tell. And you might hear someone say, "This afternoon I'm going to play golf." I started seeing the positive side instead of the negative.

SHE: My advice to other caregivers: Don't stay home and brood. Stay positive and take care of yourself, your health, your emotions, and your physical needs.

HE: I am proud to have been recognized over the years for publications and lectures in the engineering field.

Our daughter made a special trip here with her daughter from New York when I was diagnosed. She said, "Dad, even though you may shuffle and have a mask-like face, you're still you inside."

I LIKE THOSE BREAKFAST MEETINGS

AGE: 73
DIAGNOSED: 3 years
HE: Parkinson's Patient
SHE: Spouse

SHE: His voice is his biggest problem, as his speech is garbled, slow, stuttering, hoarse, hesitant, gravelly, and sometimes I can't understand him at all. What concerns me the most is that he's never going to be able to communicate with anyone.

HE: The worst part is not being able to talk. I understand very well.

SHE: About five years ago he knew something was going on. He said, "I'm going to die. We'd better have a party for our 50th anniversary." That's not like him. About a year before that, I knew something was going on, but I didn't know what it was and I didn't know how to approach it. He would get in a daze almost. At our anniversary party, he stood in the middle of the dance floor, overwhelmed, with his hand to his forehead. People who hadn't seen him in a long time noticed how different he was.

At work he was frustrated and upset because a job he was working on went wrong and he didn't know why. He was a precision grinder. Everything he did was precision. He worked on projects that had to be blown up on a screen 62 times larger than its actual size. He ended up damaging his shoulder, and he didn't go back after that.

He has to stop and think about what the next words are going to be. Sometimes he's saying he'll throw something at me, and it has nothing to do with what we're talking about. About three years ago the doctor said, "Your brain holds a lot of different words and sometimes you know the words you want to say but the brain throws out something else."

We originally started out with a neurologist. My husband said, "I don't like the way the meds make me feel." The neurologist said, "You will have to take them. Don't come back until you're ready to take them." So then we got a name and number from the support group and started going to someone else – a movement specialist.

He was diagnosed with Parkinsonism three years ago, at age 68. Somebody explained to me that there are ten or more diseases like Parkinson's disease, but aren't, and they don't know what to call them, so they group them under Parkinsonism.

My grandson found out about BIG AND LOUD (LSVT) therapy about six months ago. My husband went and was doing really well. It helped him as long as he was doing the exercises. He promised one of our daughters he would do the exercises so he could always talk to her. But he didn't keep his promise. He said, "I'm never going to get better," so he just gave up. Even with the BIG therapy, he still has a little trouble with balance, and has trouble putting one foot in front of the other.

He drove until about four months ago. He had problems before that, but he would not give up his license. It was dangerous. After he had little accidents and made several attempts to cover them up, I said, "That's it. You're not driving."

He has eye problems, but they haven't found anything when we go to the eye doctor. One eye wanders this way and one wanders that way. His skin pulls away from the bottom of his eyes. It's probably a muscle.

I was afraid of everything. I've been to every support group meeting for the last two years. I didn't think I should go if he didn't go, but I went by myself and have only missed twice. He's never gone to one single meeting. I read about it in the paper and I just showed up. I feel like they're family at the support group. I can ask questions and get answers.

HE: I like those breakfast meetings.

SHE: He wants to be home by three o'clock every day, no matter where we go.

He fell for the first time in the last three or four months, hitting the top of his head, forehead and nose, and bruising his arm, but he got himself up. He's fallen right in front of me by raising his leg trying to put his pants on.

HE: I really went down hard.

SHE: He chokes often, especially at meal time. He has to take Miralax in the mornings for his bowels. He had shoulder problems, but it was probably related to his job. It wasn't considered to be something related to the Parkinson's.

HE: What concerns me the most is that I never want to go into a nursing home. My wife is a wonderful caregiver.

SHE: At first, I thought he was ignoring me when I talked. I felt terrible because I was trying to do a good job taking care of him and I just thought he didn't give a darn. Now that I realize he isn't ignoring me, it's such a relief, even though it's still hard for me to handle the situation.

Our two daughters think the doctor should be more aggressive with treatment.

Our lifestyle hasn't changed too much because he never liked to be in crowds and he was a homebody. We really have no social life together as a couple. We may go out to lunch or breakfast, and maybe once a year we go out to dinner. We never go to somebody's house. They come to us. As of now, I'm still able to leave him alone. I bowl once a week. I belong to two 55 and over groups and I try to get to them monthly.

We finally sold the cottage we had. For 28 years he was constantly working on it. For the last five he said, "I can't take care of it anymore." He used to do everything, all the yard work and all the painting. He tore walls down and rebuilt the whole inside. Now we have to hire everything done. He has a hard time letting go.

He goes to bed at 8:10 p.m., reads for about 20 minutes, shuts the light off at 8:30 p.m., goes to the bathroom at 12 a.m., doesn't sleep well , and sleeps 'til about three or four o'clock in the morning.

Every morning he brings me my tea and cinnamon raisin toast. He'll ask – "Caffeine?" He does almost all the letting out of the dog. He mostly sat in front of the TV until he started doing word search puzzles. He gets up at 4 a.m. and does them sometimes for five hours a day.

I would advise others to exercise. Every day he does some physical exercise. But he doesn't do enough.

He was born in Pittsburg in the slums. He had a really, really hard childhood. Both parents were alcoholics. He was a beer drinker. At first our neurologist thought he had water on the brain. We were all praying for water on the brain because they can tap that. They did a test and drained the spinal fluid off the brain, and the doctor thought he'd be so much improved. Then she realized it was not water on the brain.

By age 21 he could run 21 machines in a machine shop. He's a self-made person, and did pretty well for having only a tenth grade education.

Every day I face a big challenge, wondering if he's going to fall when I'm not here, worrying that he'll get to the point he'll walk out the door and I won't know where he is.

The hardest thing for me to cope with is having to do things that he never let me do before. I was spoiled. With our five kids, everyone had a job and he and the boys took care of everything. I never made out an income tax form, never cut the grass, never painted.

Those things were a "man's job." Now I have to hire everything done.

The support group has been great for me. I don't know what I would have done without the meetings or the caregiver's support group because I didn't know anything about Parkinsonism.

Is there hope? He just gets worse all the time, but I've loved him since 1955 and I still love him.

He doesn't have to worry about a nursing home. When we need to, we'll have our daughter help out. She goes to every doctor's appointment with us as our advocate, and she keeps records of all his information.

[See his daughter's story on the following pages.]

ONCE DADDY COULD FIX ANYTHING

Daughter of Parkinson's Patient

I am his daughter, and one of his five caring children. I am his medical advocate who goes to doctor's appointments with him and my mother, and who helps make medical decisions.

My father has Parkinsonism. It affects his speech. I've not had a ton of experience with Parkinsonism, but it seems like it's affecting his way of thinking, too. He's more compulsive. He's obsessive. He tends to clean and wipe things down a lot even if you're in the process of making dinner. He comes right up to you and wipes. He does three to seven word search puzzles a day. That's his obsession.

If you look into his eyes, it's like he's looking into the distance or not looking at you at all. You're not sure if he's hearing you. It is difficult to interact with him, and it seems like we children are becoming his parent.

His eyes jump. His focus is off. It's gotten worse as time goes on. Dad noticed symptoms around three or four years ago. Mom noticed symptoms three years before he did. She noticed little things like his softer speech, and his inability to find the right words. His spatial relations and coordination has gotten tremendously worse. He was a man that did fine, tiny, intricate work, and now he's not even able to put things together that are much larger.

The biggest thing with dad is people can't understand his speech. It is more than just slurred. He has difficulty finding the words. And then when he does, he stutters. He'll use the beginning of the word and say it six or seven times before he gets the words out. He'll smile at you because he knows his brain is stuttering, but he can't get it out. And sometimes his voice comes from a low, guttural sound.

I can talk to him about events of the past and he remembers – places he's gone, places he's lived, things he did with pals when he was young. But, if you ask him things about last week, he can't seem to recall them as readily. And a big one for us is he says "no" when he means "yes," and "yes" when he means "no."

To paint a picture of my mom and dad: My dad was always the strong one and mom always came first in his life. She was an only child. She was a wonderful mother, but she always had someone to take care of her. Now she has to reverse that, and she has to take care of him. She has to make all the decisions, pretty much without him, so she now relies on us to help her make the decisions.

The doctor put dad on medication for memory, and it seemed to help for a little while, until the last 18 months. His short term memory seems to be getting worse again. Every doctor's visit, it seems to be a concern. Six months ago, he said he absolutely would not try any new medicines. He just hates all the medications. At that time, we got him to try the patch for memory. Three months later, when they did a cognitive test, like a written test, to see how his memory was, his memory had improved. One of the tests is A is to 1 as B is to 2. He has to draw a line to each. At that time, he got them all right. Before that, he didn't get them right, or would refuse to do them. They had him draw a clock and put the hands on it at a specific time. He drew the clock so small he couldn't fit the numbers in, so he said, "I could not do it." He couldn't grasp the fact that he could do it over and draw the clock large enough for the numbers to fit. To me, it seemed like he didn't realize that he had plenty of paper, and that it was within his power to change the clock and make it bigger. His signature has always been small and tight, but it's gotten very, very small and tight.

The big one for me is, they gave him a letter, and asked him to name as many words that start with the letter.

For instance, F, and he'll say, "Found, find, fine – OK I'm done." He just quits, even with prompting. We tell him he has plenty of time. He says "NO, I'm done." I don't know if it is his stubbornness of not wanting to do it, or if it's his brain just not functioning to the point where he can do it.

My father always had to have everything in its place. I noticed that when we had a garage sale, he had to move the lawnmower out of the way for it. When it was time to return the lawnmower, he couldn't return it to its normal spot. He looked at it and looked at the spot and couldn't figure out what to do.

His illness has impacted everyone in the family differently. Some are more physically and emotionally distant, and don't realize that he's not the man he used to be. I, on the other hand, feel, "That was my daddy, the man that could fix anything." Anything that was broken, whether it was a relationship or a repair, emotional or physical, he could fix it. And he can't fix it anymore. We have to fix things for him.

Though he has diminished capacity in a lot of ways, he's very aware when people treat him like a child. I'm not one to sweep anything under the rug. Some people seem to treat him like a child – even the doctor – patronizing. The problem is sometimes he just wanders – his mind wanders. But, it bothers me when the waitress looks at my mother and asks, "What did he say?" when he's sitting right there. It takes patience to wait for him to talk, so I asked the doctor what to do. She says, "try to pull his attention back to the room or the conversation."

There are virtually no emotions in his face or voice, so when anger comes on, you don't have any facial clues. He'll slap his hand down on the table, which is as much warning as you'll get when he wants to prove a point. At the doctor's office, he walked out. He felt we were ganging up on him. I find that very sad. Even expressions of love, there's no emotion in his voice – it's just very monotone.

I have a two year old grandson that's on the autism spectrum. He and my father are on the same level. I noticed it, and then my children came to me and said, "Grandpa sounds exactly like grandson, struggling to find the right words." Grandson could read at age two, but he couldn't speak. He's learning to speak, but you can't understand him. He knows what he's saying but we're in the dark. Same for my dad. I've heard people say, "I can't understand him. I can't follow his conversation."

And though mom and I saw this coming on, it still seems sudden to us. It still feels like it all happened so quickly. I do know where I get my stubbornness. I get it from my father.

It's been my experience that when we go to the doctor's office, I hear one thing, and my parents hear something else. I cannot stress enough, how important it is to have another person there to hear what the doctor has to say, and to take a notebook and write things down. There have been many times I've gone back in my notebook and found the answers to questions we have – how many milligrams dad is supposed to be taking, what adverse effects he's had from medications, what his blood pressure was, his weight – things that may come into play eventually. I've got it written down. How is his posture, how does he walk, has he fallen, why does he fall? Everything that happens, write it down. Then, you have notes telling you what the doctor said and the date she said it. I can't stress it enough – with any illness.

I believe that you should switch doctors until you're comfortable and find someone who doesn't make you feel bad when you leave the office.

It feels like dad is slipping further and further away from us. I feel like there's something we should be trying, but there's nothing new being offered right now.

Dad's not frustrated, but I am and my siblings are. We know we're losing him and we want it stopped. Dad's fixation is, when is the doctor coming, when is she leaving, and when can we have breakfast? I'm not living with him, but I see him often. The other siblings that don't see him as often see huge changes when they do. "Wow, dad's gotten really bad." If it's been a while, they might even say, "Be prepared for what you're going to see."

Probably eight months ago, my dad was doing things that would really make my mom upset. I asked him, "Dad, are you doing that to be defiant?" He said, "Yes, sometimes." That made my mom furious. Six months later, she's still very angry. I say, "Mom, he's not doing it for defiance anymore." His brain gets set when he has a thought, and there's nothing that will change that. You can say, "No, no, don't do this or don't do that." You need to get in his face, or give a physical cue to him to get him out of it, such as touching him on the shoulder or arm to draw his attention back.

My mom and dad were shopping and he had to sit down. His brain said, "Sit down right now and right here." Instead of going to a nearby bench, he sat on a shelf with flowers on it. She said, "No, no, no," because she was thinking he could have broken that shelf. Instead, she needs to take him by the arm and lead him to a bench.

He's always been a perfectionist, and is always very neatly dressed with his hair combed just right. That hasn't gone away. But when his spatial relations were off terribly the doctor told him he had to be tested by the Secretary of State in order to continue driving. He was told he could drive only in the neighborhood, but then little accidents occurred and he had to give it up altogether.

He can't multi-task.

I look around their house and see reminders of who he was and how he is so vastly different now. All the little carvings he did, and crafts he did, and the chores he did. The last thing he gave up doing was his lawn. He would spend hours on it and took such good care of it.

Mom is coping much better since she knows he's not doing things on purpose to hurt her. We can help her and say, "Go to bowling and we'll be here. Go to your evening meetings, and we'll make sure he has dinner." She needs to know that there's someone else available, and that she can say, "Oh, your dad is driving me crazy today," and that it's OK to feel that way. I'm glad she gets out. She goes to the senior center and the church to do things, and I'm glad she has her bowling. I'm glad she goes to her Parkinson's support group meetings. She needs to vent to someone outside the family. I think it's important that caregivers consider being on a mild antidepressant, because it's a very difficult and depressing thing for them to go through. Their health can be affected, too. She's dealing with this every single day. She needs to mellow out. We're afraid she's going to have a heart attack.

It's very difficult to watch and feel the person you once knew disappear before your eyes. Yet, I feel like it's our turn to take care of our parents who are growing older.

[Update: three months later]

I only wish he was as good now as he was a few months ago. He's gotten worse. He's more helpless and child-like. He can't tie his shoes anymore. He doesn't know how. "Can you show me how?" he asks.

I know there's a shadow of my father in there, but it's just a shadow. I get a glimpse of him, and then he's gone.

DEPENDING ON OTHERS – LIKE IT OR NOT

AGE: 68
DIAGNOSED: 5 years
Female Parkinson's Patient

Right now, I'm just OK. I'm slow. My balance is not as good as I'd like it to be. There are a lot of things I can't do. My home is not kept up like it used to be, but that's OK. I do what I can, and I don't worry about it like I once did.

I worry about my swallowing because my aunt, who had Parkinson's, choked to death when she was eating. They don't know whether the disease is hereditary or not. I don't know what caused mine. I don't feel like I was exposed to anything, such as chemicals, which they sometimes attribute it to.

Sometime seven years ago, one day in church I noticed my hand was shaking; a movement that was involuntary. I thought, "That's weird. What the heck is causing that?" but I didn't really think any more about it. Then one day when I was taking a nap, I couldn't turn over. That was bizarre to me. I couldn't understand why.

I didn't report these things to my doctor because I didn't think that much of it. Five years ago, I went for a checkup and my primary doctor thought I had Parkinson's disease (PD). He told me to see a neurologist. He said I wasn't blinking. I said to him, "Why do you think I have PD? I never blinked a lot." Who'd think it was so obviously PD? Now I can recognize it quite easily in someone else.

Seven years ago, during a regular office exam, I was given routine blood tests. They discovered I had Hepatitis C. I couldn't believe it, so I got a second opinion. If left untreated or the treatment doesn't work, it's deadly, so I went through Hepatitis C treatments. They have no idea what caused it. I think it might have happened when I got a flu shot in college; at that time, they didn't change needles. I agreed to be a case study for a drug company testing their first chemotherapy. It was a horrible, horrible thing and dangerous, with side-effects. During that time I was so weak and felt so "punky," I attributed everything to the chemo treatment.

When my primary care doctor told me to see a neurologist, I made an appointment, but he was not a PD specialist. He did some standard testing consisting of walking, reflexes, and strength, and said I definitely had PD and probably had had it for years. Most of all, he mentioned the non-blinking and he asked me about the tremors. When I walked I didn't swing my left arm. My writing was tiny, and I thought, "What the heck, I can't make my hand enlarge the writing." I had trouble pulling my pants up. I thought, "Why is this so difficult? It's frustrating."

I was diagnosed five years ago, two years after I had first noticed symptoms. I felt disappointed when I found out because I knew it would change my lifestyle, and it did, almost right away. I used to move fast, and pull my husband all over the mall. Now guess who's pulling who?

The neurologist told me about an orientation to be held at the Michigan Parkinson Foundation, which I attended. From there I heard about the local PD support group and my husband went with me. It was very welcoming and comfortable; I didn't feel out of place there. They recommended I go to a neurologist who specialized in movement disorders.

My medication has never been increased, since the beginning. In fact, when I changed doctors, the new doctor cut my dosage back somewhat. However, I started taking an extended release medication about one and a half years ago. The doctor probably added that because of my lack of energy, my weakness, and the symptoms that were getting more pronounced. That seemed to work OK until recently. My energy level is down again.

My posture is getting worse as time goes on. I have trouble trying to straighten it out. I can drive, but I don't.

I can't type anywhere near as fast as I used to. I was very fast. That's how I got my job as secretary for the assistant principal where I worked just short of 17 years. My former boss, a quadriplegic, was an inspiration. He taught me that humor is number one; to survive you must be able to laugh. I never heard him complain. He also taught me that I have to depend on others. It's frustrating but I'm going to depend on others, whether I like it or not.

My husband loves me and he wants to help me and protect me, but he will overdo it. The longer I can stay independent and do things for myself, the better it is for me to keep my muscles going. It's very rewarding when I accomplish things. I feel so good when I put my shoes on, and think, "Well, I did it again this time."

I'm very blessed; I married my soul mate. My parents wouldn't even attend our wedding. They eventually found out what a good man he is. We have been married 50 years. We're a close family with four children and five grandchildren.

I can't bend down and pick up the ball to play with my grandchildren, but my husband says they are the light of my life. "She perks up and enjoys them and laughs," he says. The baby is so darned cute. My three younger sisters are a good support and they want to protect me, but they sometimes hover. I tell them, "When I can't do, I'll tell you."

I don't know what I would do without my church and my faith. It's very comforting. We have the best church in the world, the best pastor in the world, and the people are so friendly.

For hobbies, I still do a little knitting. I still do crosswords puzzle. I like logic and just about any kind of game. I play simple video games. I can't do my paint by numbers anymore. I have assembled the poetry I've written over the years into a book for my kids. That's fun.

Eventually, a cure for PD is going to be found; no doubt about it.

My grandson, at age eight, said, "When I grow up I'm going to be a scientist. I'm going to find a cure for Parkinson's."

[See her spouse's story on the following pages.]

WE HAVE FUN – WE KNOW HOW TO LAUGH

Male Spouse

If someone saw her moving around, they might think there was something wrong with her but they probably wouldn't know it was Parkinson's disease (PD). The doctor spotted the masking right away, and the lack of eye blinking. I thought it was only normal aging.

I can tell her balance is bad. She doesn't like to admit it but, going downstairs, I'm always in front of her so I can catch her, or going upstairs, I'm behind her, so if she falls, I'll have her.

The first thing we noticed was her hand shaking, and her leg would be bouncing like a nervous kid in church. That's when she was on that medication for Hepatitis C. When I talked to the Hepatitis C doctor, he said the shaking was a normal reaction from the medicine because it was strong. He also said it was normal to lose one to two pounds a week. She lost 50 pounds in over 48 weeks.

We were both always hyper, doing something – babysitting, or running around. She tries to do that now, but she can't; her reactions are slow and she just gets too tired. It takes her time to answer questions, too. I have to sit still and wait for her reply. Her body is fighting Parkinson's all the time, but I think the medicine tires her, too.

She stoops and she shuffles. I take her shoulders and try to bend them back and push on her hips, and ask, "Now, doesn't that feel good?" Drooling was one of her first symptoms, but she didn't know that years ago when she got cracks on the sides of her mouth from drooling during the night.

She has rigid muscles and cramps in her thighs and calves. Her voice is very low and quiet. She has to take high fiber food because the medicine causes constipation. She gets mad that she can't button her buttons. Her handwriting is small. I wash her hair. We take our showers together. I used to have to cut her meat, but she seems to be able to do that better now since we added a medicine.

She used to love baths. She made a habit of relaxing in a bath while I took care of our four kids. Now she can't get in and out of the tub; she loses her balance.

When I retired, they called me back to work to run classes. That was the best job, but after five years I told them, "I can't do it." I couldn't leave her at home alone; she's a little paranoid. Anything we did, we did together. She woke me up one night because she couldn't breathe; she couldn't get enough oxygen. I called the ambulance. They said, "We've got to get her to the closest hospital." They said it was caused by stress and worry.

She gets vivid dreams. I just hug her.

It's hard to accept her limitations. She's willing to do things; she just can't because she's always tired. We used to go to the recreation center and walk the track and go swimming. She can't wear shoes because of toes that are bent. She can't even ride the bikes. When she was really bad, I had to take her in a wheel chair. Then when they gave her a 24 hour slow-release pill, there was a huge difference in her overall energy – she was staying up longer and was more active. It made a major difference for a couple of years, but now I can see that she's going back to how she was.

I get my support from her. When I help her, she knows I'm helping her and she appreciates it.

Her big thing is playing cards. If she could, she'd play seven days a week. I'd just as soon sit in a chair in the living room watching a football, baseball, or hockey game.

Whenever I help her, I leave something for her to do. I think she might hurt herself if she does too much more than she does.

The biggest challenge is mostly fatigue – endurance. She was very self reliant; she could do anything. She's paranoid that she won't be able to do things for herself if I'm not here to help her.

We met in junior high, swimming. I was diving. There was always a lineup at the diving board. She was my public leaning pole. She was little and cute, so I'd prop my arm on her shoulder, being cool. She was probably the best thing that ever happened to me; she probably kept me out of jail. She had a sense of humor, and we were always laughing.

As a caregiver, I remember that as husband and wife, we took a vow for better or worse. With me, there were plenty of times I was sick and she had to do all the work, so now it is payback time.

We're both on the right side of the grass. We have fun. We know how to laugh; you have to laugh at life. Words that I try to live by: Have a good time whenever you can. For us, we do everything we can together.

The prognosis is not good. Better medicine is needed. They've got to figure out something to correct the problem. It's going to continue to get worse. The medicines are just a delaying mechanism to slow it down. Maybe Parkinson's doesn't kill, but it can lead to death because of complications of the disease. Her aunt, her mother's sister, died of Parkinson's from choking to death. She was elderly, living in assisted living because her husband couldn't take care of her anymore.

Michael J. Fox had DBS for one side of his body. It was terrific. He could cut down on meds because of it. Then the symptoms started on the other side. You have to continue to increase the meds for the symptoms to be controlled, but there are a lot of side effects.

We promised that once the kids were raised, it would be time for us – if we wanted anything, we would get it. And then, the grandkids came along...

DON'T GIVE UP THE SHIP

AGE: 76
DIAGNOSED: 5 years
Male Parkinson's Patient

This disease is making me old before my time. Since I've had Parkinson's, I look much older than I actually am. I have tremors, and am slow moving and slow responding. I have stooped-over posture. My tremors, of my hands, and occasional spasms of my legs, are very bad. They will just start jumping until my meds kick in.

Everybody tells me I have masking. People see me and say, "Have you been ill?" But what I see in the mirror doesn't reflect much change.

Drooling is not excessive, but it does occur. It could occur anytime.

If I sit for two to three hours to watch a movie, I need a crane to get me out of the chair. I find that on many occasions, once I do get out of the chair, I have to concentrate to get in the upright position to start taking the first step. After that's accomplished, I can get going, but the gait is much slower until several steps are taken. When the medication is at a high point, I walk at a normal gait. If it's not, my gait slows down.

My voice is becoming much softer. It's lower in volume, automatically, where if I wish to speak in a rougher, louder, tone, I have to exert energy to purposely increase the volume.

I have a tendency to lose my balance and I have to take two or three steps backwards to stop myself from becoming a person with broken bones.

I have to drive because my wife doesn't. We don't go out as much as we used to. I'm very cautious to drive the speed limit, and in many cases, below that, for better control. I very seldom drive at night, due to possible cataracts on my eyes. Starbursts from the headlights of the oncoming automobiles temporarily blind me. It won't be too much longer that if we want to go somewhere, we might be walking.

I kept the diagnosis of Parkinson's disease (PD) from my children for a year because I didn't want to put undue bearing on them until it was absolutely necessary. It wasn't a case of I had leprosy or anything, but there was a noticeable change, which the children caught onto very quickly. When I finally did tell them, they said, "We knew it anyway." I was seeing something different in the mirror than they were seeing. I didn't see the obvious.

I do choke, but I'm not so sure Parkinson's has anything to do with it. I say that because if I have a piece of candy, I end up coughing, choking, sneezing, and it goes on for two minutes. It brings tears to my eyes. It's scary. Other times, I'll be sitting there eating dinner, and we call it, "It went down the wrong pipe." When it occurs, it's almost a mirror image every time.

We were told that my handwriting would trail off. "Your writing will become smaller, and it will trail off up or down." That's exactly what happened. I start out normally, but then everything goes uphill, and it trails off and gets smaller and smaller and becomes a straight line. How do I take care of that? I don't write very much.

My words will trail off, too, because I lose my train of thought and can't finish my sentence. However, if I wait for a period of time, it comes back to me and then I'm able to complete the sentence. I'm embarrassed and frustrated, because I know the thought is there but I can't get it, unless I'm patient and wait for it to come back again. By then, the point I'm trying to make is lost. Memory loss is getting worse as time progresses. I guess I've got the beginning of Alzheimer's, being that I'm almost 80.

I was around 71 years old when I went to my regular doctor for a yearly check up. He noticed that my left hand was beginning to shake. I called it "shakes," he called it "tremors." He said, "I want you to go to this neurologist," which I did, reluctantly. The neurologist gave me tests and said, "You have Parkinson's disease." I said, "I'm not so confident that you're making the right diagnosis. I'm not sure I have Parkinson's. I'm going to get another opinion." He became indignant and said, "OK, go." So I went to another neurologist, a movement specialist. He said I had the first stages of Parkinson's. The first neurologist had put a cap on my head, with little pins or nails in it, and it would press into my skin. And then he had gauges that would jump and turn like in the old time movies, to see if I had Parkinson's. After a half hour of that, he did a reflex test on my knees. Doctor number two asked me where I had been, and what had I discussed. "How come you didn't like him?" he asked, meaning the first doctor. When I told him what I'd gone through, he said, "There is no test to determine that a person has Parkinson's, except to monitor the patient over time." So I immediately had a lot more confidence in this doctor than I did the previous one, who must have thought I was a guinea pig, I guess.

My new doctor started me out with medication, though a stronger dosage than I take now. We lowered it because of side effects of hallucinations. I was violent, fighting off my wife, thinking she was another person attacking me. I never got out of bed, or attacked her. It was always just grabbing her, shaking her with a lot of strength. Then I started seeing things in my peripheral vision. If I look at an object, I may see something different than you. I may see a boat sitting in my driveway, or some people camping at the bottom of my driveway. I'm in the process now of cutting back on my meds. I'm knowledgeable enough to know that it's only me hallucinating and that what I see can't be real. I've learned to ignore a lot of things I see because I say, "That's not possible." When I'm driving, I assume that what I'm seeing is real, for safety sake. It occurs day and night, but not all the time. When I get violent, it's always at night when I'm asleep. I talk in my sleep. It's incoherent. My wife tells me, "You were talking to somebody."

I say, "OK, doctors, you've been working on this Parkinson's for who knows how many years and you haven't found a solution yet." So I get angry that we haven't made more progress than we have. What does it take – twenty billion dollars to solve the problem? It's all fine and dandy, making improvements. What's stopping us from accomplishing the task of finding the cure?

I've been involved with Parkinson's for five years, and the only thing that's changed, to my knowledge, is I'm getting progressively worse. That's nothing new. And I don't mean to be critical of the efforts put forward to all concerned. I become frustrated with what comes back from these tests that are being worked on.

I participated in a drug trial for a year. Someone was suing the manufacturer of a medication for possible side effects. Extensive exams were performed by the doctors. They were saying the medication was OK.

I exercise every morning, floor exercises, and I lift hand weights.

I have to keep track of when I took the last pill so I don't overdose. Or, I forget until I think, "Oh, Oh, I should have taken it," because the juice is running out of me. I very slowly shuffle over to the pill box and take what I should have taken 45 minutes before. It takes 20 to 30 minutes for the medication to become effective again.

The future is very bleak because I have a disease that is not curable, and eventually down the road, I will become a burden to the rest of my family. I guess it makes me angry. With Parkinson's, we take the medication, but every month it gets worse, with no cure in sight. It's difficult to have positive thoughts when you know the end results are disastrous. The only thing we can do is the best we can.

I'm more dependent on my wife for ordinary functions, like assisting me to put on my coat. Very seldom does she help me dress. If we're in a hurry, I should have started 30 minutes earlier, because I can't get my arms in my sleeves. I can do it, but it takes three or four times longer.

When I was first diagnosed, I could do anything I wanted to do outside and inside. Over the past five years, the periods of time I can work without resting are becoming progressively shorter. I get tired. No climbing ladders now either.

I've continued to golf, but it's getting progressively harder to play the game. I can't play as well as I used to. I'm going to attempt to play this coming summer. Swinging the club correctly is the hardest part. And of course, there are hundreds of jokes about golf to endure.

What helps me cope is my family: seven children, and eight grandkids, and our friends. We go out to dinner, to a movie, or play cards. The PD support group helps both the patient and the caregiver share and sometimes solve day-to-day problems.

I have some depression. When the day is sunny, I feel better.

I have given up thinking that everything has to be done at this particular moment. We don't get excited if one of us misplaces something. We'll say, "It'll show up tomorrow or the next day." We're a little more tolerant of errors that occur unintentionally.

I was born in Detroit, on a kitchen table at home. I have a brother and we're 16 years apart in age. I met my wife when she was five years old and just starting school. She lived a couple streets over. I went to school with her brother. She just tagged along with everyone else. We decided to make it permanent when she was 19 and I was 20. They had the draft then and I had to go in some service. I went in the Marine Corp. After I got out, we got married. After I retired, I travelled around the world, doing consulting. My wife got cancer, and I quit consulting. She's the one that has helped me most in coping with this disease.

[See his spouse's story on the following pages.]

WE HAVE TO HAVE PATIENCE

Female Spouse

I noticed his hand was shaking. We used to sit in the living room and read the paper and have a cup of coffee. After a while I said, "Why is your hand shaking like that?" He said, "I don't know." It got worse and worse, but none of this was affecting our life, really.

We had gone to Arizona so it was probably in the winter. My sister in Arizona noticed it. I said, "Yeah, I've seen it." When we got back home, I said, "We're going to see a doctor." The first doctor just said it was tremors but gave him all kinds of tests and told us to come back in a year. It got worse and worse and my husband said, "I'm not going back to him." That's when we went to a neurologist who was a movement specialist.

He walks a little bent over. His arms don't swing like they used to. He takes smaller steps. He used to take longer strides and bounce when he walked. He doesn't do that anymore. The hardest part to accept is the change in him. He's not the person he used to be.

He was having really bad nightmares. When the doctor finally changed his meds, I told him the change was a life saver. They cut back on one medication and gave him another that he cuts in half and takes only at night when he goes to bed. He doesn't have those nightmares any more. They were violent; he would hit me in his sleep. He hurt me a couple of times. Finally when I'd get him to wake up, he was always chasing someone, defending himself, and he'd grab me on the arm. It's not fun. He was doing that for a couple of years. It's not his fault; he didn't know what he was doing. I told the doctor about it a couple of times. He just said it was a reaction to the meds. I don't know why it took them so long to change them, but they did, and this is the third week on different meds. He stills sees things, but the nightmares have stopped.

We did most of our travelling before he was diagnosed; we went a lot of places all over the world. Since he's been diagnosed, we've driven down to Arizona a couple of times. However, we've been flying for the last four or five years, and we keep a car down there. This is the first year we haven't gone. He also has a back problem and a pain in his leg. They're testing for nerve damage. He has arthritis in his spine. It's not Parkinson's related that we know of. It just compounds the problem.

I try not to hover. I probably do, but he needs help sometimes, and I think he's beginning to accept that more, like putting on his winter coat. The hardest part is trying to watch him get dressed. It takes so long, but I hesitate to help, unless he asks me, because he wants to do it by himself. I think he tries to do more things than he's capable of. Saturday he got on a mover's truck to try to help someone move. It was slippery and we had to talk him into getting down.

When we first got married, I worked. After the second child, I didn't go back to work until after my seventh child was age eight. I worked for two years as a receptionist at a toy company.

His Parkinson's hasn't kept me from doing anything I like. I like to travel; I enjoy that a lot. We play cards. I collect snow babies and music boxes. I really never had much time for hobbies and activities with all the kids. I was a big reader, but I can't do it anymore because of my eyes. I have diabetic retinopathy.

For support, if I have a bad day, I can talk to my friend; her husband has been diagnosed with PD, too. And the Parkinson's support group is very informative.

I would advise other caregivers to have patience. Try not to do things for them. Try to encourage them to do things for themselves. Wait for them to ask for help, even if you think they need it. I think if you do too much for them it becomes easier for them to not want to do it anymore.

Sometimes when the meds aren't working as well as they should, everything he does is so slow, I want to do it for him. You just have to hold your tongue. You want to finish his sentences, or do it for him because you can do it so much faster.

Probably, I put my own well-being on the back burner sometimes if there's something he needs, or the kids need.

I have faith that everything will turn out for the good.

I WANT SOME ANSWERS

AGE: 52
DIAGNOSED: 6 years
SHE: Parkinson's Patient
I: Mother and Caregiver

She was diagnosed with Parkinson's disease (PD) about six years ago, at age 46. We noticed that every once in a while when she would reach for something, her hand would shake. We didn't make a big deal about it because we thought maybe she wasn't feeling well. Her sister had her over to her house and later asked me, "Did you ever see her with a tremor?" I said, "Yes." The family doctor gave me names of two different neurologists. I called one and they set her up for an MRI and a brain scan. He said, "She has Parkinson's." I asked, "Well, what do I do?" I had no knowledge of Parkinson's. He said, "When the tremors get really bad, bring her back and I'll put her on meds." I asked for a written report. "It doesn't sound right," I said to my primary doctor, "Why do we want to wait until things get worse?"

The doctor agreed with me. She said, "The report doesn't seem like it's thorough enough." So I went to a second neurologist and I took a copy of the report with me. They tested her, said she had Parkinson's Plus, and put her on Parkinson's medication. I said, "I don't understand what that means." He said, "There are other things going on in the brain," but he didn't explain it. Then I began going to the Parkinson's support group meetings, which I had seen listed in the paper. I spoke with the leader. She gave me the name of a female neurologist who is a movement specialist, and said, "Maybe she'll work out better for your daughter."

The second neurologist did brain wave tests. I didn't know if what they were telling me was right or wasn't right. My poor girl was born mentally challenged. She has a congenital heart defect – a hole between her upper and lower chamber. When she was born, 52 years ago, doctors wouldn't touch a mentally challenged person with a ten foot pole. At that time, I was told she wouldn't live to see her teens.

When people first see her, they know that she's mentally slow by her lack of response. She always appears to have a serious look on her face, and she's kind of in her own little world. She's not very vocal. If I have something important to discuss, I have to sit her down, make sure I have her attention, and explain to her what is going on and try to get some feedback from her.

She doesn't have a loud voice. I can't hear her in her regular conversation. We went to a voice class at the hospital rehab center – LSVT. It is a great class, but she hasn't continued using what she learned.

She was fitted for hearing aids but she won't wear them. She's always thinking about something else, mostly music. She plays music, "In my bedroom," she says. She plays piano, too, in the front room. She's had almost ten years of piano lessons.

Before she had the Parkinson's, she was more alive, more interested in life. Up until two years ago, she was able to work six hours a week at a local chain restaurant. She worked in maintenance. She had been at New Horizons where they found her the job. They selected her because she was higher functioning and she wanted to work.

She worked at the restaurant for ten years. She loved it. Life was very full for her. Two years ago she kept tripping and falling. She fell at work, and the bus driver told me that she fell.

Now, sometimes she's too tired to do things she used to do, like bowling with her friends once a week. When she gets up, before she can get mobile, I have to massage her head to toe. We do some leg exercises, because sometimes the legs don't want to move, even with the walker.

After we take care of her in the bathroom – washing up, and relieving herself – she wears adult diapers – we exercise with weights, with a band, and with a ball. We do sit-ups to get the heart rate and the circulation going. We do it at home. She wouldn't do it on her own.

Her tremors are not a consistent thing. They're on and off. When I ask her, "When do you think you have tremors?" she says, when she's excited and talking to someone. Her hands go a lot. To me, it seems like she wants to say more and speak quicker than the words want to come out.

She trips. The brain and feet are not coordinating together. Her feet want to go faster than the brain. I'm with a lot of special needs people because they're her friends. I can tell they're trying to tell me something, so I don't interrupt them. I can see they want to say, "Wait a minute – I'm not finished talking."

Sometimes near the end of the day, she will drag her feet. If she sits a full hour, her legs are so stiff she has a hard time walking. If I'm home, I'll make sure she gets up more often to use her legs.

She had two bladder infections within a two month period. She doesn't listen to signals in her body that tell her to empty her bladder all the way. Her urologist gave me a letter saying, "She needs an expert that has other tools and devices. I'm afraid all I can do is prescribe meds." A neurologist/urologist spoke at our support group and I made an appointment with him. He hooked up an InterStim to her bladder. Since she's had this procedure, I cannot leave her alone. Before that, I was able to. It's a trial period for three weeks before they can implant everything inside of her. When the bladder gets full, I have to take it off. She said she wanted it on because she was tired of wet pants. It's hard trying to get her to understand. The doctor said if she didn't have this done, and continued to have bladder infections, it would affect her kidneys.

I asked my doctor, "What does Parkinson's Plus mean?" The doctor just said, "It's complicated." I want answers. Nobody gives me enough information. I want to know what's going on with my daughter. I'm her caretaker. I want to have as much information as I can to give her a good lifestyle. This is why I go to the Parkinson's disease support meeting. The doctors aren't telling me, and I want to hear from the average person what I can expect. Sometimes you get more information from average people than you do from the doctors. I keep a day-to-day diary. I'm going to show it to the doctor next time I go. Otherwise, they only listen to what they want to hear.

My daughter's case is unusual. She lost the sight of one eye due to glaucoma. Every time I turn around there's something going on with her.

The worst thing with Parkinson's for her is the incontinence. It's not just the bladder, it is also the bowels. And now she's working with a goiter. The doctor put her on medication to help relax her bowel. I didn't see it helped any, and she said, "I don't want to take that." The urologist reviewed her meds and said, "I don't think she should be on this for her bowels." He said it also stimulates the bladder, and that's why she's wearing these adult diapers because her bladder is leaking all the time. That was about three months ago. We took her off that. I think there's been a slight improvement of the constant bladder drippings.

She has never driven a car. She has worn glasses since she was about two years old. We use eye drops everyday for her glaucoma. If she lives long enough, she'll probably have to have a fake eye, which is a lot to take care of. She sees her eye doctor about every six months.

Every once in a while when she wakes up, she'll say, "I'm shaking, I can't stop shaking." I'll see her body going. Sometimes it's only one leg.

She was in the Special Olympics and in field and track. She never swung her arms. When we would go walking, before her walker days, I'd say, "Swing your arms." But she never did. When she was born, her elbows were out so it's her bone structure. In the 1960s, when she was born, the doctors just put a tag on special needs and nobody researched any further. I went to a geneticist who thought she had cerebral palsy, but all the tests came back she did not.

I didn't understand the PD diagnosis at all. When I started to research on the computer, I thought, "I'll do whatever I have to do." The PD itself hasn't changed my life – but the effects of the PD have. I don't feel comfortable leaving her. I worry about her falling if I'm not here. Sometimes I ask my other daughter to watch her so I can get out of the house. I don't do that too often.

I thank God I'm a healthy 75 year old, but I am concerned about the future, wondering if she's going to outlive me. She can't be by herself. She falls in front of me. She broke her wrist last summer, not using her walker, and she had to have her wrist in a cast. If she does outlive me, her sister says she'll care for her, but she has a husband and work schedule that might not allow her to do that.

I've been widowed 25 years. We had seven children. My children are not too far away. My husband always felt, "The more the merrier." Nine was not enough. We had ten or eleven people around all the time. To go from that to just the two of us, it's lonely and sad. Sundays are the worst. I'll take her to the library or we'll go somewhere. The kids say Saturday and Sunday are the only days they have for themselves. Half the kids don't come over to visit anymore, and the grandkids are away at college.

We used to go out more, to concerts, and to the theater, but now with her bladder problem, we just can't. I'll just have to wait and see if this will help. We used to go for walks every day or to the parks. Now, if we go for a walk with the walker, she'll tell me she's tired or her legs hurt. In the better weather, I walk every night after dinner while she's watching her shows. I try to ride my bicycle often. I have to get out of the house at least once a day.

I'm a person who accepts what I'm dished out and I just try to make the best of it. Being a religious person, I know I'm not going to walk this journey alone, and the other thing is, where will it get me to be angry? I pull myself up by the bootstraps and say, "Handle the situation as it comes up. Move forward. When you're in a pity party you're by yourself."

I love being around people. I used to volunteer at the school and the senior center. I always enjoyed dancing. My husband and I used to go to dinner dances all the time and we were always up and out on the floor at weddings. I enjoyed being a wife and mother.

Now it's her and me to face the world.

IT'S A COMPLICATED STORY

AGE: 69
DIAGNOSED: 7 Years
HE: Parkinson's patient
SHE: Spouse

HE: I really don't even think about how other people see me. For me, I do what I can, so I don't want to sweat the little things – the slowness or the softness of speech. I don't think it's that important. My problem is not with my movement, it's with my short term memory.

SHE: If anyone interacts with him for five or ten minutes, they will know he has Parkinson's. He's slow with his movements and speech.

HE: I've slowed down quite a bit, and my voice is softer. I keep searching for words...

SHE: except when he's talking about things he's really interested in. When people talk to him in a way that demands answers, he is slow, because he's searching for answers. Everything is in slow motion, including the movement of the head. Masking of the face has come and gone.

It's a complicated story. Seven years ago, they diagnosed him with Parkinson's and put him on medication. He was still working. Everything was fine, and the medication helped with the slowness of movement and masking. But it had side effects, and the medical and pharmaceutical establishments do not talk about side effects.

He became hyper-sexual. We had no idea that it was a side effect of the meds until a relative of mine said, "Do you think it is the meds?" I went on the internet and found that, indeed three percent of those taking this medication had side effects of hyper-sexuality, gambling, shopping, and eating. He had the hyper-sexuality. When we shared this with the doctor, he said, "Oh, yes, this medication could have that side effect." Five years ago, he changed the meds. Everything seemed great. Then I noticed a few things, but thought it was my imagination, so I didn't express my opinion. However, I didn't understand it. My husband was trying to control his sexual urges and was feeling very agitated. Three years ago, it came to my knowledge that the hyper-sexuality was still going on. I didn't know until we had a huge upheaval in the house, and again searched the internet, that the new meds had a two percent chance of side effects of hyper- sexuality, too. The doctor didn't tell us that statistic either. It became very difficult for my husband to control those urges. Six months ago, our new doctor stopped all his meds and the urges went away. We've talked about this so much, and been through so much. It has been very hard to deal with.

Doctors don't talk about the side effects. I discovered the statistic because I'm inquisitive and dig into things. The British websites are much more informative and open about how the side effects of certain medications contribute to compulsive behaviors, and how lives have been affected because of it. They're extremely candid and lambast the pharmaceutical companies. There was a guy in England who sued the pharmaceutical company and got eight million dollars. While he was on the meds, he had started gambling and lost everything.

I'm incensed at how it's upset our life. The doctor's reaction was, "I agree. We can decrease the meds a little a bit, but this is the minimum he can be on." The problems continued. The doctor said, "It's such a small amount, it can't be the meds," and he didn't take him off it. The doctor's response was a very big disappointment. After his meds were decreased, the doctor checked my husband's motor skills and said he was doing fine on a lower dosage.

My husband was trying to control his hyper-sexuality, but even with the smaller dosage of meds, the feeling was still in him. We were so frustrated with the doctor because of his inconsistencies that we changed doctors. The new neurologist looked at his history and said, "We need to take you off this medication." I haven't seen that behavior since the medication was stopped altogether six months ago. Now the only meds he's on are an anti-depressant and one for alertness.

The man that I knew before this medication cloud sort of came back. The masking, to a large extent, was no longer there. I felt like he understood that I wanted the best for him, which made it much easier to communicate and work as a team. Before that, he had paranoia that was directed at me – thinking that I was spying on him and that I was doing things to make his life miserable.

The new neurologist, a specialist in movement disorder, thought he had Lewy Body dementia, and thought his was not classic Parkinson's, but Parkinson's syndrome. She did neuropsychological testing, an MRI, and blood work, and we'll go back next month for results.

HE: I retired four years ago, after 36 years, and am Professor Emeritus of Political Science at the university. I'm working on a book about politics in Kenya where I was born. I left there when I was 21. Before I retired, at school, I was able to walk four flights of stairs. I've been trying to do that – keep in shape. We walk at the senior center a couple of miles nearly every day, except weekends. Exercise helps tremendously. I took six or eight sessions at the BIG and LOUD physical therapy.

SHE: It was wonderful.

HE: I do the exercises every day. I believe in it because it makes such a dramatic difference when I walk. In the morning, when I get out of bed, I'm stiff and achy. After the first exercise I feel OK. I do my BIG exercises and my muscles loosen up. I don't even have the limp I had before I was exercising. I have huge problems with writing and I can't type anymore really.

SHE: It's not that he can't, but it takes him a lot longer because he can't remember where the letters and numbers are on the keyboard.

He's fallen three – four times out of bed, and I don't understand because he's so slow and not jerky in his movements. We have an adjustable bed now that is helpful.

HE: I'm too stiff to get up after sitting awhile.

SHE: He counts one, two, three, and rocks so he can get up. He's very tentative the way he walks or sits down. They say it is fear. He drives, but he doesn't drive far. He'll go get gas, or go to the university, or to the drug store.

HE: I drive during the day, not at night because of the lights of the oncoming cars, but I still feel that I am OK on the road. My wife is much more sensitive about it. She'd rather I not drive.

SHE: The doctor said a couple of years ago, that he had mild dementia. Then six months later, he said he had moderate dementia. Then later, an aide did the testing. The doctor read her notes and said, "He doesn't have dementia." I knew that wasn't the case. My husband and I were so open and detailed about what we shared with the doctor, so he had plenty of information to make a more accurate diagnosis.

At night, my husband takes two meds for hallucinations. The good thing is, the hallucinations don't scare him, but he's irritated by them. He has had hallucinations for two years. He now sees people during the day. He sees mostly silhouettes.

HE: During the day I see youngsters following me around. They're just milling around; they're not threatening. They're just fixing a door – but it's not like they're attacking me. One time, at night, I told her to turn on the light and they disappeared. That helps me to distinguish between what's real and what's not.

Occasionally, just suddenly, my nose will drip.

My dexterity has decreased. I have drooling during the night. I can shave, but I'm slow and I don't shave often enough because it takes so long. I have a goatee and mustache. I have no problem with my appetite.

SHE: He has trouble with his fine motor skills. He's not as efficient, like cutting with a knife, or putting a shirt on with buttons.

I don't think he eats as much as he used to. He loves sweets. He didn't used to at all. His sense of taste has been dulled. He's been using more spices than he used to. I think that's why he likes sweets; he wants something with more intense taste. He lost his sense of smell a long time ago. He chokes easily; two out of five times that we sit down to eat, he chokes, or if he's drinking something, he'll choke.

HE: I get tired very easily.

SHE: We go out and we try to be back for him to be in bed by ten o'clock. He has expressed, within the last couple of months, he doesn't enjoy big happenings; he likes small dinners with friends. We don't go to loud parties any more.

HE: I've enjoyed going to the symphony concerts. That's a different kind of loud.

SHE: If we do two things in a day, it's exhausting for him. He doesn't like a lot of conversation.

HE: That's what tires me.

SHE: Four years ago he was on meds for prostate problems; he was in a fog and couldn't remember anything. That's why he retired. We happened to go to a Parkinson's disease seminar. Our movement specialist was the lecturer. He mentioned that one of the meds that was contraindicated for PD was the one that my husband was on. We saw the neurologist and he cut out three meds that the urologist had put him on. When my husband came off those, he was fine, but two and a half years ago, the dementia resurfaced. My advice is, do your own research.

I didn't think the Parkinson's would be such a huge thing. I thought we'd do the meds and just deal with it. The side effects had a devastating effect on our life. I would ask my husband why he was doing what he was doing. When you have a fight about something like betrayal of trust, even when you know it's the medication, the kind of feelings that get eroded can't be repaired completely even though you understand it. Pre-dementia, my husband was a very, very smart man and he would argue convincingly about his point of view. If he had recognized that it was the meds causing the sexual behavior, he could have said, "This is not who I am." But, the sexual feeling is a very good feeling, with a lot of good energy inside. You don't want to give it up. He was never able to accept that it was the medication. I knew that it was, or I would have divorced him, obviously. It's really damaged my relationship with him. We're doing the best we can.

The side effects have resolved themselves. Right now, we're contending with the dementia. At times he understands he has dementia, and at times he doesn't. I know it's increasing. It's too overwhelming for me to think about the future. I think about today, and how I can make life better for him today.

I need to concentrate on taking care of myself, too. Right now, I'm in the process of taking over the finances. I haven't pursued my hobbies. I try to meditate; I exercise. I have support from my friends and family. My children have been very supportive. I always try to carve out sometime during the day just for myself. I listen to music and read. I like to paint and I like to garden. The PD support group has been very good.

My fear is for his safety, that he will hurt himself. Right now, he has a bump on his head from falling out of bed. I don't get angry but I get very frustrated. I know he tries, but he just can't do it. Sometimes I feel he's just not trying hard enough, though. I'll say to him, "When you sit in a chair, you pull the chair out, you get in front of it, and then you pull it to the table." We practice sitting down, but he sits on the edge of the chair, partly because his spatial perception is off. And he places his plate always off. He doesn't space himself correctly. I ask him, "Why do you do that instead of doing it right the first time?" He feels like it's too much trouble, or I think he just doesn't remember. It's the same thing over and over. He thinks I'm nagging, but I have to keep reminding him, even in the same moment. It's so much effort even to do the simple things like that.

I put his meds out for him in a pill box because he was making mistakes taking it. Now it's not complicated for him since I have them measured out.

I worked for medical research labs before I worked as a school psychologist. I was also a clinical psychologist for adults. I did testing and worked with behavioral problems. My background has helped a lot both in psychological and biological understanding. I think it's a complicated disease. If you don't understand it, you look on the surface, and think, "He's just being difficult."

We both retired four years ago. I retired then because he was in a fog due to the prostate meds and I really couldn't leave him at all. We thought he had to go into assisted living. At some point now I think he might have to go into assisted living. It's a concern, because he hates the idea. We've talked about it; at some point I won't be able to take care of him. Right now we're managing pretty well.

We have two children. They've known about the Parkinson's from the get-go. Their relationship has been complicated since three years ago when they found evidence of his hyper-sexual activities that he carelessly left around. They came to me and said, "Look what we found." I was shocked. Later, when I found out his problem had to do with the medication, I told them. It was very hard for them to think their dad had done all this stuff.

I feel burdened, so that's why I have to take mini-vacations, a respite-type of break. I go away with my girlfriends for the day. I'm really "it" – the only one taking care of a lot of things in the house. He used to be a full partner.

No one in his family has had Parkinson's, but he used to use Roundup® very freely, without a mask, and without gloves. I'd say, "Why don't you wash your hands?" "No, no. I don't need to do that," he said, but now Roundup is [allegedly] linked with Parkinson's.

The support of my family and friends has been incredible and my kids and I are very, very close. They've seen how difficult it has been. Anyone dealing with Parkinson's should get as much information as they can to understand what's going on. Go to the support group. Someone there will know what you're talking about. Don't rely just on what the doctor is saying. Do your own research. Talk to others going through the same thing. The hope is, you do the best you can and maybe they'll come up with drugs that don't have such devastating side effects.

I KID YOU NOT, THERE'S A SNAKE ON THE FLOOR

AGE: 74
DIAGNOSED: 7 years
HE: Parkinson's Patient
SHE: Spouse

SHE: His shoulders and head are starting to stoop over and I can hear his leg dragging when he walks. He uses a walking stick which helps him straighten up a little bit. His hands are starting to curl in; so are his feet. He stares a lot. He's looking younger, though, because he's lost weight, for one thing, and his face looks more relaxed.

HE: The tightening in my shoulders and back causes me to be bent over. I stumble sometimes. I fight it, but the trouble is I don't even notice these things happening.

SHE: The year before he was diagnosed we were walking the beach with his brother who said, "You've got a little shake in your hand there. What do you think it is?" We just assumed it was his heart medicine, but a year later, the shakes were getting worse. Our primary doctor said, "I think you should see a neurologist," and he gave us the name of one. The neurologist put him through a bunch of tests, and he diagnosed my husband with Parkinson's disease (PD). He was a terrible doctor, though. He never answered his phone, and never returned calls. That was six or seven years ago.

HE: About four or five years before that, we were climbing a mountain out west where the dinosaur remains are. I was climbing and doing fine, and all of a sudden I couldn't move.

SHE: He was petrified; he sat down on a rock and said, "I can't do this. I just can't do this." I held his hand and he slid himself to the bottom. It was sad.

HE: I really didn't know what PD was when I was diagnosed. The doctor said, "We'll see you in six months." I thought, "This can't be too serious." In his office was information about the Michigan Parkinson Foundation. We went to one of their regular orientation classes held for people who have symptoms or questions about PD. There we learned about the PD support groups.

SHE: Going to the support group opened our eyes to the different stages of PD. Neither one of us knew how serious it could be. We get a lot of important information; information about exercises and about drugs that are coming out.

We met our doctor when he was the guest speaker at our PD support group. He is a movement disorder specialist. I like him because he's blunt and doesn't sugar coat things. The subject of night terrors came up. My husband and I looked at each other. He had been having night terrors for years before he had other symptoms of PD. We didn't know what they were. During the night in his dreams he would start shouting, thrashing around, hitting, and shooting people, and I would be on the other end of it. I'm a heavy sleeper, but I would wake up with him screaming in my ear. They were very scary.

One time he had the flu. He couldn't get out of his chair and I couldn't pull him out. He got on the floor and tried to turn himself around. It took him probably an hour and a half to crawl into the bedroom because he had to keep resting. I was going to call the kids but he said, "No, I can get in bed." He had taken a cold remedy, and that's the only thing I can think of that would have caused that condition. He literally was like mush.

He used to be a social butterfly and an outgoing salesman. We went to a social Sunday and when we got done eating, he said, "We have got to go." He mentioned it about five times. He was uncomfortable.

He's more timid now, his speech is very slow when he tries to communicate, and, like right now, he's mumbling.

HE: I don't realize I am. My voice is soft and it's slow; I think I'm speaking up when I'm not. I lose my train of thought easily.

SHE: We built a business for our livelihood; we have three. My husband was a dynamic business man. He doesn't come across that way anymore. He gets very anxious and nervous if he has responsibility. He gets afraid to talk to people; he acts like he doesn't know what to say and his thoughts don't come out right. When he's talking, I say, "Don't mumble. Talk louder. Bring your voice up." Now when we have a business meeting, people talk to me and talk down to him.

HE: Business was always my hobby. We started a hobby business for retirement. It has become pretty active. My wife didn't want to get involved. She just wanted to have more grandchildren, but when I started to slip, she started making sure the business stuff got done. She has been really supportive. We're both licensed builders. We have been listed in the top ten builders in Michigan. In the past, I have been real active politically and socially, but now I've resigned from those things. I'm not doing as well as I used to.

SHE: He's slow at anything he does anymore. I'm always saying, "Come on. Hurry up." I think he gets absolutely exhausted and he can't lift his legs. We went out for a walk. By the time we were getting close to home, he was tired and was leaning on me. He couldn't straighten himself up, and he couldn't make it any further. If alone, he would have toppled on his head. That's what happens when he gets tired. That would have been a cake walk up until six months ago.

His vision has gotten very bad over the last four or five years. I don't think it's related to PD. He's been going to a cornea specialist and a retina specialist. He has

Uveitis, a retina disease. He started getting shots in his eyes.

Other things we notice: He'll be eating, and all of a sudden this little bubble, just one drip, will appear on the edge of his nose.

HE: I don't drive because I'm afraid I'll fall asleep. It could be dangerous.

SHE: I've been driving for about nine months.

HE: Sometimes when my arms tremor, you can't see the tremors, but I can feel them within myself. I'm slower in doing things with my hands. My writing starts out normally, but ends up getting really tiny on the end.

SHE: I can't read his writing. Basically all he writes now is his name. I've noticed he's starting to have trouble with his knife and fork coordination. He was struggling to cut his steak when we were out at a restaurant last week.

HE: I can't carry two cups of coffee at the same time because I shake so much, but the left hand doesn't shake too much. All I want to eat is sweets. If you sat me down to ice cream and cookies, I'd be happy with that.

SHE: He'll go, "I don't want these vegetables; I don't want that; I've had as much of this as I want." But 15 minutes later he'll want ice cream. His desire for sweets is unbelievable.

HE: I can't smell anything. It's been a couple of years. I don't know if it came from PD but it must have. I drool a little bit at night. Metamucil® is a staple in our home for constipation.

SHE: We asked for the patch because he was falling asleep all the time. The doctor said he was too old for the patch. I think he falls asleep because he's totally bored and doesn't have anything to stimulate him. He was asleep on the couch the other day and woke up shouting, "I kid you not, there's a snake on the floor." In the last six months, things like that happen to him.

HE: So many people don't know anything about PD. When you have something like this yourself, it's pretty obvious to you when you see it in someone else. I looked at two of my friends and said, "You've got Parkinson's." They said, "No, No." Sure enough, when they went to the doctor, they found out they did.

SHE: I try not to worry about the future; otherwise I'll just get depressed. Last week at that party, I had a man come up to me and say, "I just want to tell you my brother has Parkinson's and my sister-in-law had to put him in a home. Don't ever feel bad if you have to put him in a home. He'll be better off." We have four boys. I don't think we'll ever get to that point.

HE: I'm very fortunate that we have a large support group. We're blessed with good family and friends. Our kids are all supportive. We have four boys, fifteen grandchildren, and ten great grandchildren, ages two to thirty three. They're all close by; within a 20-25 minute drive. Everyone kind of molds their situation so it's comfortable for us. During the week we normally go to games; we go to basketball games and soccer games, baseball games and football games. They make darn sure grandpa is taken care of.

SHE: They watch out for him. They help me out with his appointments, which gives me a break. I call my grandchildren my heart medicine. They relax me and keep me from getting discouraged. I spend a lot of time doing crafts with them and they put on shows for us.

HE: I'm really happy to be alive. I've gone through a lot of crap. I try to find the positive in everything, and enjoy life, but I have been wondering about the death situation; how my wife will be. We've been married 48 years.

SHE: All of a sudden he's been thinking about what's going to happen if he dies. It makes me sad. He gets anxious about it.

HE: I haven't found PD to be a challenge at all. I know Parkinson's is going to win, but I don't dwell on it. Socially and family-wise, we run all over the place. I can still do what I've always done. I can't do it as quickly.

SHE: Whether he wants to admit it or not, our life is changing. As caregiver, I'm doing everything I've always done plus doing everything for him. Before, I could ask him to run to the grocery store. Now he can't. We used to go camping. We've camped all over the U.S. We've been in every state except Alaska, and about half of Canada, and have travelled with our family all over the world. We still travel, just differently.

Most people don't understand, by looking at them, how bad a person with Parkinson's is, or if they do, they don't say anything.

HE: My wife has not only been supportive but she's done many good things. She's on the board of a foundation that we've endowed with a scholarship in both our names – a scholarship for kids who want to go to college or a trade school, just as long as they're going into the building business.

SHE: We've been very much involved in charity. We believe in giving.

HE: We volunteer to do anything and everything.

SHE: He used to enjoy helping me cook. Now, I have to dice the onions myself. He was 6'5". He's shrunk. I no longer have to stand on my tippy-toes to kiss him.

CLIMBING THE NEXT MOUNTAIN

AGE: 75
DIAGNOSED: 7 years
Male Parkinson's Patient

I am stooped, I have a masked face, and I shuffle when I walk. The masking of my face came about gradually after I was diagnosed with Parkinson's disease (PD). I have significant problems with balance, freezing, and with overwhelming fatigue. My stooping has become more pronounced in the last three or four years, as has my shuffling.

I was diagnosed with PD seven years ago. I probably had it as early as 13 years ago or even earlier. My wife says I had it much earlier, perhaps before 1976 due to my gradual loss of smell at that time. I have since heard that the loss of smell is often the first indicator of Parkinson's. For the last 13 years, I have had pronounced stiffness in my legs whenever I would sit for a period of time. Around seven years ago, I had a right arm tremor that I had incorrectly attributed to wrist problems, and to the wrist surgery and bone removal that I had. I was probably ignoring the symptoms.

I was 69. I already had a very good neurologist for my Myasthenia Gravis. At one of my regularly scheduled appointments, she, along with her partner, suggested I had Parkinson's because of a lack of arm swing on the right side, and because of right arm tremors. I was upset because she made light of it, not really telling me what the diagnosis meant and confusing me when I asked her if the symptoms could be controlled. She said, "Absolutely, well controlled," which is not really true, especially in the later stages. She also prescribed a medicine that was ineffectual. I was overwhelmed – emotionally and physically. I got a second opinion from a movement disorder specialist, a well-respected local doctor, who she referred me to at my request. We had a few tense moments discussing the issue.

I wasn't a very happy camper with the diagnosis of Parkinson's, once I began to understand what it meant. I had had a really bad year, with a whole list of ailments – glaucoma, and a serious G.I. bleed (I lost 11 units) when hiking in the mountains of Tucson, where I almost died. And I had a diagnosis and treatment for prostate cancer. All that, as well as my right wrist surgery.

The symptoms I have right now with my PD are significant. I have overwhelming fatigue, freezing, and problems with my balance, although my balance is improving with my exercise program. They are my major problems. I have freeze-up moments constantly. I count, or grab an inanimate object close by, or use my hiking stick – anything I can to break the locked position. To march up and down while turning slowly seems to work also. It's hard to turn around without falling over. These symptoms limit me and what I can do. They get worse if I get upset, nervous, have a crisis, or have an argument with my spouse. My symptoms seem especially sensitive and driven by my emotional state, so, I try and stay calm.

Other things I deal with are: I have excess saliva during the day, but few problems drooling, except very slightly at night. I have the typical voice problem – I talk in a soft, raspy monotone. I limit my driving. My digestive system is slow. Two prunes a day mostly solve that problem. My nose drips when I eat. I have upper back problems. I have problems with hand-adeptness. I have good days, and less good days, and it's hard to predict what it will be. I used to be a good typist. Now I struggle. My handwriting is small and illegible. Brushing my teeth is a lot easier if I use an electric toothbrush and a flossing tool. And, of course, I have my various other health issues, with their associated symptoms.

I don't have a real problem cutting meat, but I have my wife do that for me occasionally. I also have what's called REM sleep behavior disorder, (commonly known as RBD) which causes vivid dreams that are physically acted out – a reaction to one of the meds I'm taking. (I had switched to it, as another one I was on caused dyskinesia, and was otherwise, ineffective.) I fell out of bed and physically reached for my spouse as if I were chasing her. I have a medicine now that controls that issue fairly well by calming the brain down at night.

To be pro-active, I got involved in the state and local Parkinson's support groups. I sought out experts and information by talking to people, reading, building a good reference of key books, and by trying to be a keen observer of what was going on with me. I went to the library, checked out Amazon.com, made a commitment to continue to exercise, and got engaged in the PD community. I worked on the Walk/Run for the Parkinson Foundation. I've continued to be active in the PD community, and with the local support group. The support group provides me with invaluable information, inspiration, education, and emotional support. I go to seminars with my spouse. She's been active in the local Caregivers support group.

I have three important ways I deal with the disease: I go to a competent movement disorder doctor, I have an exercise program to do every day, and I learn as much as I can. I've taken a very aggressive approach to learn as much as I can. I had a two-page list of questions when I first talked to the local support group facilitator, and I got good, solid answers to all of them from her. I started working my program right away, upon diagnosis from the second neurologist, and have continued to be diligent in dealing with its issues since. I advise you do that, rather than be passive, nonassertive, and apathetic toward the physician, exercise, and information.

I consider the changes in my life due to PD as challenges to be met. I will admit that the balance, freezing, and fatigue problems are kind of overwhelming. They really are. They provide a constant challenge. My choices are kind of limited, as far as what to do about it. My doctor brought up DBS surgery two or three months ago. "I don't have anything else in my tool kit," he said. I probably don't qualify, as the risk is high, and I have many other ailments and procedural and medication related risks associated with them. And, it won't help my balance, fatigue, or freezing problems.

I retired before I was diagnosed with Parkinson's. Even though I had been diagnosed with Myasthenia Gravis 16 years ago, I continued to work until I retired ten years ago. I worked in facilities engineering for an automotive company, and was involved in many related utility, rate, legal, and regulatory aspects. After I retired, I worked as a consultant for some three years, on two very complex and very successful projects in Mexico.

Following my diagnosis of thyroid cancer, I started running. I went on a vendetta to run to scare the cancer away. During the next 20 years, I ran several marathons and triathlons, did many long distance bike rides, and went on several mountain treks in the Alps in Europe. A year after I was diagnosed with PD, I did a 26 mile run/walk with over 5000 feet of ascent and descent in Pennsylvania. I finished standing up.

I exercise daily by walking on a stair machine, using the elliptical, treadmill, and stationary bike machines, and I do the occasional five mile shuffle run, supplemented by weights and balance routines. I try and spend at least ten to fifteen hours a week on my exercise program. I try and fit in the LSVT routine once a week also.

We attend the symphony, chamber music concerts, and the local symphony. We have a home theatre set up for movies and TV.

I am an electrical engineer, and hold three degrees: BSEE, MSEE, and MBA, and am a licensed professional engineer. I was a torch bearer for the 2002 Olympics, representing my department at work, in Akron, Ohio. The selection was based on position, education, and my disability at the time – Myasthenia Gravis. I retired from my company at the highest technical (non-management) level available in 2003.

My spouse is struggling with the demands my disease makes on her, and the things I can't do. She also has her own health problems.

My best advice is to exercise habitually; otherwise it's of limited value. Get a good doctor. And learn all you can about the disease. I also think one of the best ways of coping is to deal with the moment, not the past or the future.

One of the things that bothers me is we get lectured by experts who don't have Parkinson's. That's one of the reasons I've been involved in the orientation meetings at the Parkinson Foundation. Another thing that bothers me – there is not a lot of emphasis on the role of the caregiver, and what they have to deal with. To our facilitator's credit, she's set up a monthly caregiver's support group, in response to a suggestion. It's well-attended, and a place where caregiver's feel free to share.

[See his spouse's story on the following pages.]

WE WANT TO GIVE BACK AND HELP OTHERS

Female Spouse

I remember him talking about having problems with his vision. He went to the doctor. The doctor sent him to a neurologist who diagnosed him with Myasthenia Gravis. That was 16 years ago. Ten years later, the neurologist observed him walking down the hall and said, "I think you may have Parkinson's disease (PD)." The doctor noticed that he walked with a particular gait that is common to PD.

My husband didn't like the medication the neurologist gave him from the beginning. He couldn't eat what he wanted to with it. Somehow we found out about the monthly PD support group meeting. We went to our first meeting in November of that year. I can remember thinking, "Thank God this year is almost over," because between us, we had about five health issues. I had a brain aneurism. He had gone to Arizona and fallen on cactus while hiking with a friend. He had needles all over. They spent a day trying to pull them out. We were still pulling them out over a year later. The fall could have been due to PD. It was only months later that he was diagnosed with it. He has not had a sense of smell since we moved here in 1975. I say he's had PD since then. I think the disease moves at different speeds for different people, depending on the situation, or stress.

At the fist support group meeting we attended, we heard about a neurologist – a movement specialist. He's been going to him ever since, and he's been very happy with him.

This disease has affected the quality of our life, and there are constant changes. He doesn't have the physical ability to do things, so I'm doing things now that he always used to do.

His change in appearance has been very gradual. The curve in his back was there before we were married in 1965. He's never been one to smile and have a quick easy grin. He doesn't have quite the chatter he used to have before PD – it's harder for him to speak. He is not quite as outgoing as he used to be.

One thing I'm kind of sad about is, we can't take off and go where we want to go anymore. I was looking forward to our retirement being a time of exploration. We used to look forward to a drive out west every year, planned by him. We went to the mountains, camping and hiking. Three years ago, he said, "Let's go to Alaska." We made plans, but we had to cancel that trip because of his problems falling. However, we are going to the PD conference this year in Michigan because someone else is driving. We don't socialize like we used to. Our circle of friends has dropped way down because he can't stay up late.

I have learned, during this whole period, to rely on the third step from the 12 step programs, which reads, "Made a decision to turn our will and our lives over to the care of God as we understood God." It makes a difference for me to know what I can do, and what I can't do…and to learn to accept what I can change and what I can't change. It's helped me in regards to living with someone with this disease.

While in the Navy, he started doing the Royal Canadian Air Force exercises every day. In addition, in the 80s, he started running. And then he started biking. I started biking, too. I couldn't go as fast or as long as he could. He used to be able to ride 100 miles a day. He hiked, in Europe, mostly, and met people there that he's remained friends with. He has exercised all his life in hopes that he'd have a healthy life. He can no longer hike, bike, or travel.

His fatigue gets worse every year. If he's had an exhausting day, he'll spend the next day in bed sleeping. About two years ago he started freezing, which occurs when he's walking and tries to turn around.

When he was first diagnosed with Parkinson's, he had trouble putting on his jacket. I tried to help him. He got angry and said, "Don't help me. I want to do it myself." I said, "I won't offer to help you unless you ask for it." And that's what I do. Now I will reach out to help him only if I see he has a problem. I've heard other Parkinson's patients say, "I want to be independent as long as possible." Now he is at the point where he'll reach out his hand if he needs help. Sometimes he needs help getting up from a chair.

We each have our own pill dispenser for the week. He takes his own medication and orders both our medications. It gives him participation in his life and mine.

Our PD support group system is like an extended family. I've had a couple of women come up and say, "If you need to talk, here's my phone number." I'm not used to help being offered me. I've been on my own so long. We are both only children, and we don't have extended family nearby.

We met while we were both in college in Chicago – he, at the Illinois Institute of Technology, known for architecture, design, and engineering. I was studying art at the Art Institute of Chicago.

The best thing I've done for myself has been to go back to university as an adult. I got a Masters of Fine Arts in theatre design and directing. I was a member of the university theatre in set design. I learned so much, and gained a lot of self-confidence. It's helped me deal with our health issues, as it's given me a sense of what I'm capable of.

I love music, concerts, and live performances. I love our cat. I love painting. It keeps me young and sane, and gives me a legal "high." I am taking a class in needlepoint, and water colors.

The hardest part for me to accept about his health is watching the disease progress, knowing that I won't always have him with me. He was really good at his job and what he was doing. I'm very proud of what he accomplished in his career in engineering in the auto industry.

I would advise other caregivers to take very good care of themselves – their inner self. And to find something that they absolutely love to do that takes care of their soul.

My words of inspiration that I live by: "To thine own self be true." If you aren't true to yourself, how can you care for your loved one? I think a lot of people, through care giving, can end up with a lot of anger and dislike, and may penalize themselves or others. The caregiver's health is critical – their mental, physical, and emotional health.

To stay married to someone for 48 years, you have to learn to be a little flexible. And we try to live with what comes along day by day.

I think our Parkinson's group is phenomenal. I'm glad we have it for the support and care and love we get, and hopefully give to others.

We participate several times a year in our state Parkinson foundation orientation meetings as guest speakers. We feel it is one way we can give back.

DON'T STOP THINKING AND DEVELOPING

AGE: 76
DIAGNOSED: 7 years
Female Parkinson's Patient

My family can always tell when I'm tired because my face goes blank. I notice it in photographs, too. I used to have a wide, vivacious smile. Now I don't smile as often. I must look drawn, because they ask if I'm tired.

My balance is bad. That bothers me more than anything else. Sometimes when I get tired, I can't get my muscles to move at all. They lock. I just sit there until I get the message through. My speech is affected sometimes, too. I slur. It just comes and goes. I think fatigue is a trigger for me. I take time-released medication. I can tell when I'm due to take it.

My handwriting becomes very precise but very cramped. I probably print better than I ever did in my life, but not all the time, and it's very tiny. I have weakness in my right hand. My posture is poor compared to what it used to be. That bothers me a lot, as I used to be so upright from my dance and my skating training. I spent my youth skating. I started at age seven and skated until I was 23. I skated competitively in the U.S. and I toured Europe with Holiday on Ice. I went to Russia for three months in exchange for the Bolshoi Ballet.

I was very active. I did yoga, walked every day, and played golf.

I'm self-conscious. I don't feel like I'm well-groomed any longer. I really don't have any interest in dressing. I have to be very cautious about that or I would tend not to get dressed every day. It would be just as easy to stay in sweats. That could be attributed to the fact that I no longer have a partner to keep me interested in doing daily activities. My husband, after open-heart surgery and 42 days of convalescing, passed away eight months ago.

Stooping just happens and sometimes I can't control it. I just bend from the waist sometimes. One day my posture can be perfectly normal and I can walk around very briskly. And, the next day I get out of bed and can hardly move. I shuffle. From time to time, I use my cane just for support to give me security.

If I didn't force myself to be physically active, I think I could become quite lazy. Fatigue is my biggest foe. I try to have a nap every day. Fatigue is definitely a problem. I feel it now. And, I'll have difficulty walking across the street by the time we're done here.

I have leg cramps periodically, which go up the sides of my calf. My feet cramp – the toes curl on both feet. In fact, they're curled all the time. My hand looks bent and tilted to the right, and there's no strength in it. I was checked for rheumatoid arthritis, but I don't have it. My right big toe is bending over the second toe. I went to buy a pair of shoes the other day, and I had to buy a pair of wide shoes with a rounder toe because of my toes bending. It looks like I have a bunion. The neurologist looked at my feet the other day and he said, "It is par for the course."

My neurologist recently did an MRI on the brain to rule out anything other than Parkinson's. They did some physical testing for my balance, like having me fall backwards, put one foot in front of the other, walk down the hall, and turn several times.

I drool at the corners of my mouth occasionally at night, and mostly when I'm experiencing fatigue during the day.

I have freeze-up moments, mostly in the evening when fatigue sets in. I'll be sitting on the sofa watching TV and I'll want to go to the kitchen to get refreshments. I freeze and it takes at least 15 minutes to take myself out of the chair.

I lose volume in my voice as I get tired.

For no reason at all, I fell sideways the other day and I went right down on the floor. It just happens. I find myself navigating through a room, and staying close to a wall or furniture for security.

I haven't driven for three months – since my brother asked me not to. He wants me to get a clearance from my neurologist.

My balance comes and goes. When I lie down, the room goes around very quickly with dizziness. When I'm walking, it ebbs and flows.

I'm doing much better getting in and out of bed since I've learned to maneuver my body. I have a way of putting my left knee up first and then pulling my right knee up until I'm kneeling on the bed. I maneuver my body onto the side and then to a prone position. I've learned to pull my right elbow back so I can roll over on my side. When I first developed Parkinson's, I couldn't turn over at all. I have trouble getting on and off the commode. I've learned to put my feet securely on the floor before attempting to stand.

My bowel movements are irregular, when I used to be very regular.

I have lack of grip and I have a difficult time opening jars and bottles. I don't have the power that I once did to wash my hair. I use a round brush with a handle on top to wash my hair.

I use eye drops in my eyes all the time.

I have an electric toothbrush now because I just didn't have the strength to brush my teeth. For a long time, I couldn't floss my teeth. Now I use a Waterpik®.

I had my brother put in safety bars in the bathroom.

I find myself using more and more salt because I don't taste any flavor in the food. My appetite comes and goes. It's periodic. I think I've lost weight because I don't cook like I did. I'm trying to force myself to cook.

My sense of smell is not as acute as it once was.

I was having trouble swallowing pills, but that's gone away. I never know when it's going to happen. Everything seems to come and go.

I used to have hallucinations when I first started on my medication. I would see animals and people standing alongside the bed waking me during the night. My dosage was adjusted, and I don't have them any longer.

I get a feeling of depression, but I think that has a lot to do with losing my husband, losing my dog, losing my house, giving up my job. We were living in California when my husband died. Two months ago I sold my house in five days. It all happened sooner than I expected. I wouldn't have given up my job if I'd stayed in California.

Six years ago, I was undergoing treatment for non-Hodgkin lymphoma cancer. I was undergoing chemo treatments. I started developing dizziness and weakness and my toes were curling. My doctor sent me to a neurologist to make sure that it was not solely the cancer that was causing my difficulty. Now, I'm completely cured of the cancer.

I was diagnosed with Parkinson's disease (PD) when I was 70. I was surprised at the diagnosis because I hadn't heard of any Parkinson's in my family. When the neurologist first diagnosed me, I asked how he could tell. He said there's not really a blood test – we tell by your actions, by the way you walk, your handwriting, and other physical tests. He put me on a mild form of the medication. I went to the computer and found out as much information as I could. I was curious. I didn't know what Parkinson's involved. Then I went to UCSF (University of California, San Francisco) where they have a Parkinson's disease department. I joined their program and saw the neurologist every three months. I attended seminars and support groups. I was terrified because the first seminar I went to, I saw all the people in wheelchairs. I decided to keep as active as I possibly could. I think mental attitude has a lot to do with how you feel.

I followed the doctor's orders in taking medication and was trying to keep my gait from dragging by forcing myself to walk more normally.

My Parkinson's symptoms didn't affect my life too greatly because I continued working. I worked with my husband. We were both in retail our entire life. We met at the J. L. Hudson Company 51 years ago. When we retired, we both became merchandisers. We both travelled in our careers to San Francisco. We loved it there. In 1997 we said, "Let's do something different." So, we said, "Let's try California for a while." We were in San Francisco for 12 years, until his death, which brought me back here to Michigan to be near family.

When I knew I'd be coming back to Michigan, I went on the computer and found out about the Michael J. Fox program at Henry Ford Hospital, the West Bloomfield Campus. My niece is a nurse there. I asked her if she knew any neurologists involved with the program. She did and she made an appointment for me.

After my husband died, I came back to Michigan anticipating the family gathering around me. But, I found out they're busy with a life of their own. I have to find a new life and new interests, and now without my husband. I never realized how much I depended on him. I have two stepchildren and five grandchildren. The stepchildren are very attentive and they're all like my own.

I can't be as active as I once was. I'm going to take a trip in May for a reunion, and I'm going to see how that works out. Last time, I swallowed my pride and had wheelchair assistance at the airport. It's stressful enough travelling.

I'm without my car right now until I get further go-ahead from the doctor and my brother. My brother hadn't seen me in a long time. He was surprised at how my physical actions were more difficult, more halting, and that's why he took the car away. I must be a lot slower than I was, because people tend to do things for me that they didn't do before.

I'm fearful of the future and what's going to happen. I anticipate, if this gets worse, I might have to go into assisted living sometime. I'm not happy about what I see for possibilities, and yesterday the investment counselor kept emphasizing how expensive it is and how fast your money disappears.

My posture and attitude are my biggest challenges, trying to keep optimistic about the future.

I love to read. It's my favorite pastime. It's the thing I do when I can't sleep at night.

I do a lot of note taking and a lot of planning. To pamper myself, I wear my husband's wedding ring. I wear my husband's prayer shawl. A group of my friends in L.A. knitted the shawl and prayed over it and enclosed a printed prayer and sent it to him when he was in the hospital.

I think my emotions are more acute because of loneliness. I was accustomed to spending all my time with my husband. We even worked together. I miss my dog. I left mine, a standard poodle named Redford, in California. He is beautiful, and his new family loves him. I can't get another one. It's too hard for me to walk a dog.

I want to attend the local Parkinson's support group. I'm concerned about the future and I want to know more what the future will be like. I'll try to learn from other people's experience, and I'd like to form new friendships.

Any advice I may have would be to keep active. Don't become melancholy. Don't stop thinking and developing. Continue living.

I find it hopeful that they're making great progress and Michael J. Fox and Mohammed Ali, among others, are looking for a cure.

BE A FIGHTER – KNOW YOUR OWN BODY

AGE: 70
DIAGNOSED: 8 years
Female Parkinson's Patient

Eight years ago at age 62, I noticed, when washing my hair, my little finger didn't always move. I felt something was wrong with my body. It felt uncomfortable and I was very tired. Sometimes when I drove in the car, my right leg shook for a moment. So, I went to my family doctor and he sent me to a neurologist. He was not a specialist, but he did all kinds of tests. He checked me from head to toe. I told him, "I have a feeling I have Parkinson's." I am a nurse and, of course, the doctors don't like it when you mention your own opinion. He came to the conclusion, "No, you don't have Parkinson's. Come back in a year." During that year, I still felt like there was something wrong with my body. When I wanted to stand up, I had to hold on because I felt weak and tired, and I didn't have the strength in my legs. I waited the year and went back and told him I didn't feel good, that I had anxiety about the way I felt. You know, I am still angry at him because he asked me where I lived in Germany, in Stuttgart. He wanted to talk about where his Mercedes was made.

I asked him, "Is there no medicine or nothing you can give me?" He said, "All these medications have side effects." He sent me home. He treated me like I was overly hysterical or overly exaggerating. I went back to my family doctor and told him the neurologist didn't do anything for me. They were friends, the two doctors. I felt really anxious and uncomfortable. I said to him, again, "I don't understand why there's nothing that can be done." The primary doctor threw up his hands and said, "You have to go to therapy." He gave me the name and address of a psychologist. I made an appointment and I got a real nice therapist; she was very understanding.

"I tell you the truth," I told her, "I am not here because of psychological problems. I have the feeling I have Parkinson's, and the doctors don't believe me." In addition to that, my family doctor had already sent me to a neurosurgeon because I had problems with my right shoulder. I've heard that shoulder problems are one of the signs of Parkinson's, too. He had several x-rays done and found a disc problem in my neck. He wanted to do surgery. I told him, "As long as I know that I don't for sure have Parkinson's." He made a remark and said, "Don't make a mountain out of a molehill," and sent me to his own physical therapy business on the same floor. I went six or eight weeks. For a while it helped.

I brought it up again, "Don't you know anybody who knows about Parkinson's?" He said, "Yeah." And, he sent me to his brother, who was a neurologist, located in the same building. I told that doctor my problem and he made me walk up and down the hallway and did the reflex test on my knees. He said, "No, you don't have Parkinson's." He's the one that needed a psychologist, he was so weird. By then I had been to a family doctor, a local neurologist, the neurosurgeon and him – four doctors.

At the beginning, when I started to question my health, I bought two books about Parkinson's written by Dr. Abraham Lieberman. I still probably have the papers in that book with phone numbers to the National Parkinson Foundation and the Michigan Parkinson Foundation. When I called the Michigan Parkinson Foundation, they told me that someone was going to start a local support group soon, and gave me a phone number. I called one of the facilitators and she told me, "Yes, I know of a neurologist. My husband goes to him." That was the second time I had heard of that doctor. So, I said, "Yes, I must contact him." That's how I found out that there are doctors that are "movement disorder specialists." I was shaking, but I don't have tremors. I was just nervous. He did some tests with me. He said, "You are smarter than all the other neurologists you've been to."

I think I was the only person who was happy to hear I had Parkinson's, because I knew I could finally get some help. Thank God. He heard my prayer, because somebody finally gave me a name of a doctor to see, to find out what was happening to me.

He started me on medication, with smaller doses at first, building up gradually. At that time, I had anxiety and depression. After six to eight weeks, the anxiety, and depression went away. He put me on an additional med, combined with that one. Three years ago, he cut down on the first drug, and I still take the same dosage of the other. About four years ago, I participated in drug trials. I discovered I did so much better on it, the new brand name, rather than the generic, which I had been taking.

I have had bladder infections two times, and I have very bad constipation. He said use senna tea. That helps. Both are problems associated with Parkinson's. The small fingers shake, and I have shaking in the right leg on the gas pedal. My right leg was so unstable, and it didn't stay quiet. I have anxiety issues with Parkinson's and sometimes I feel that inner nervousness. I get tired easily. I started having problems with my back 1 1/2 years ago. I got more tired and had problems standing up. I also notice it when it is time to take the next medicine.

Every once in a while, I think, "I hope I don't end up where I cannot get out of bed, or walk, or cannot move, especially since I turned 70 last year.

I was working as an emergency nurse and surgery nurse when I came to this country 25 years ago from Germany. My husband worked for an automobile company. To learn the language, I worked at a German bakery for some years before we got transferred to Michigan. Then I thought it was time for me to go back to nursing.

We met in Germany when he was on a business trip. We've been married 25 years. I was 46 when I came to this country. We have two boys and one granddaughter.

I hope that because I have a light version of Parkinson's, it doesn't get any worse and that I won't have to be dependent on somebody to take care of me. I still feel fine. I feel good enough. I listen to my body, and I do whatever I can to strengthen my muscles. I go to physical therapy and I do all the things I like to do. We travel. We live on a wooded lot, and I like to work outside. I go to church. I read. I meet with friends. I go three times a week to do water aerobics.

From the beginning, I was there when the monthly Parkinson's support group started.

When it comes to your body, you are the best one to know when there's something wrong. If you want answers, you have to be persistent, and not give up. I called everywhere and I asked around until I finally got help. You have to be your own advocate and be a fighter.

The hardest thing to cope with is that I cannot go on forever. I have to accept that I get tired.

The medicine and the PD doctor and the support group have helped me the most. My husband says it does not cause a problem in our relationship. He doesn't have to be my caretaker. I would say to others, just stay positive. Tell yourself you still can do what you want to do. Be thankful for that. I'm thankful that I can get out of bed every single day.

WE'LL WORK IT OUT TOGETHER

AGE: 71
DIAGNOSED: 10 years
HE: Parkinson's Patient
SHE: Spouse

HE: I look like a grouch. I don't smile as much as I used to. I struggle to talk and I start with the shakes because I try too hard. People may see me walking around with the shakes, but nobody has really walked up to me and said, "I see what you're going through," or singled me out and identified me as someone with Parkinson's disease (PD).

SHE: Our friends noticed his face before he was diagnosed. We went on a trip with them two years in a row. Someone said, "He's not smiling." So then, I compared pictures from both trips and saw the difference. The first year he was smiling, the second year he wasn't. He had that stone face look.

HE: My appearance changed. Instead of smiling, I looked like I was off in another world. I really didn't think I looked that unhappy, but it looked like that in the picture.

SHE: Outward signs he has are the mask, the tremors on the left side, and the voice. I would complain to him that he wasn't talking loud enough when he'd call home from work and leave a message on the recorder. I couldn't understand him. He just said it was a bad connection. But, it happened more than once.

HE: To me, I thought I was talking loud. It makes me self-conscious. It makes me feel like I'm falling apart.

SHE: He's great one-on one, but in a group, he just sits back in the corner and doesn't engage in conversation. If I see him with the guys at the bar, he's just sitting there. He doesn't even realize he doesn't talk. I'll make a motion to him with my jaws. He knows I mean, "talk."

HE: Instead of pushing myself, I just sit back. Every once in a while I get a day when I try to project my words so I don't stumble and stutter, but the biggest part of the time, I go around mumbling.

SHE: He's been for voice lessons.

HE: I know what it takes to project, but I get indifferent and crawl back into my hole.

SHE: He knows what to do to get the most out of his voice, but he chooses not to. He took the LSVT LOUD program at the hospital. He learned to reach down into his diaphragm and take in a lot of air and project his words out.

HE: My doctor said my stammering is just part of the stage I'm going through.

SHE: He's bent way over. A couple of times after he came out of a massage, he was standing straight. I thought, "Wow, it's nice seeing him this way."

HE: I have a hard time forcing myself to sit up, or even walk straight, or stand straight. If I know I'm going to be standing for a while, I put my hands together behind my back to force myself to stand up. Strapping myself in the seat belt in the car keeps me straighter.

SHE: He's still curled over. He walks like he's not real secure or stable. He bends over all the time and his balance is off. He shuffles.

HE: I find myself using the handrail more often. I think it's because of fear of falling.

SHE: He has drooling, mainly at nighttime.

HE: Some of the problems I deal with are drooling: I'll put a clean hanky on my pillow because I drool, and it sometimes ends up stuck to my lips. Writing, I start off and it's very big, but by the time I get to the end of the sentence, it's very small. Sometimes I can't make out my own scribbling. Driving, I start getting real tired and find myself going from side to side, wandering. It makes me feel like I'm daydreaming. I think my eyes get really tired. I'll pull over to the side of the road and let her drive.

I had scar tissue on my eyes and they had to remove it because it was working its way to the pupil. I have trouble getting in and out of bed, and turning over. I have to sit up in a sitting position in order to turn over. There've been a couple of times I've tried to get out of the chair, and it's hard to get my legs to move. When trying to put my shoes on I have problems. I can't get my foot to slide into my slippers. I have to kick it against the wall for force.

I go to the exercise center and ride the bike five or six miles and I work with the upper body weights. I do it because ...

SHE: ...because his wife says, "You have to exercise." I keep hearing that exercise is good to keep your body up.

HE: Plus it helps keep the cobwebs out of the mind.

The doctor noticed that my arms don't swing when I walk.

SHE: He'll hold his left arm, like there's something wrong with it.

HE: My sense of smell kind of went downhill right about the time I was diagnosed. There were times she would pick up on a smell I was not aware of. All our life, it was just the opposite. Now, the room has to be filled up before I can smell anything. I have trouble cutting my food. I struggle, but if it gets too much for me. I ask my wife to do it, which doesn't make me feel good. I can turn any meal into an all day affair.

SHE: He has problems with choking.

HE: Another annoying problem is that my nose has always been dripping. When I blow my nose, I have a tear running down my left cheek. When the shaking starts, I get frustrated and have an upset feeling on the inside. There have been times I go to grab something, or reach in a container to take out some jelly beans, and it seems to take a long time to grip them in my fingers on my left side.

SHE: He needs to take a little more control of his eating. He eats an unusual amount. He eats until he gets uncomfortable. He just had a hernia operation. We think he's straining too much to eliminate. He'll eat a good size meal, and within five minutes, he's into the snacks.

HE: I'm finding that anytime between two and four in the afternoon, I set myself down for 15-20 minutes. I slow my pace down and kind of get my second wind. The thing that gets me down at times is not knowing why my body shakes, or does its own thing. I feel like I'm losing control. It may be a reminder that I need to take my pill, or sometimes it may be because I'm just trying to do too much. I usually tell myself to keep going instead of stopping.

SHE: Prior to his diagnosis ten years ago, he would reach for his wallet, and he was shaking. That's when I said to him, "You know, we're trying to get things ready for retirement. You've got to take care of yourself." He made the effort to get to a specialist to see what was going on.

HE: When my hands started shaking, she'd ask, "Don't you realize what's going on?" It was out of my control, so I was in denial. I'd sit on my hand, trying to get it to stop. When you see someone shaking like that, you want to reach over and stop it for them. The first neurologist ruled out Parkinson's and told me I had a stroke. I walked around for about a year but things were not getting better.

SHE: I said, "If you'd had a stroke, you would get better." Instead, he was getting worse. The shaking was bad. A cousin was over who had a relative with Parkinson's, noticed his shaking, and thought that was what was wrong with him. I said, "We were told by the first neurologist that he didn't have Parkinson's." So then we started all over and went to a second neurologist. We walked into the room, and the doctor said right away, "You have Parkinson's." I said, "No, he doesn't. We were told he didn't. We had blood tests and everything saying he didn't." He said, "You can't tell by blood tests. You have to go on the medication, and if it helps, that will affirm it is PD." So he put him on a new drug that had just come out.

HE: When I got the diagnosis, I wasn't enjoying going to work anymore anyway. So, when they offered me a package, I took it. Basically, the way I felt at the beginning of my diagnosis was, "Well, I'm going to fight it. I'm not going to let it get me down."

SHE: We went to the third doctor to get another opinion, and then we found a Parkinson's specialist and went to him to make sure we were on the right track. He said, "Yes." He changed his medication.

HE: It was scary to hear I had PD, but I was thankful I wasn't being told I had cancer. People have been known to live a long time with Parkinson's, so I felt I still had a long way to go. Once I understood more about it, I realized Parkinson's wouldn't kill me, and that I'd probably die from something else. However, when I started noticing others with PD, it was depressing to see some of them in further stages. I wondered, "How soon will I be going through these different changes." And then, some of the people were no longer with us. My doctor said there are five stages. I'm at the second or third stage, and if five means being in a wheelchair, I don't want to be there. I want to keep moving as long as I can.

SHE: My friends noticed how he was shuffling out to the mailbox. He'll shuffle and stop right in the doorway. We don't pay attention anymore, because we're accustomed to it. He's been doing it for four or five years and he has fallen. He probably didn't bring up his leg far enough. However, we're not experiencing a lot of falling.

HE: I have to make sure I look ahead in the direction I'm walking.

SHE: He's moving slower, he's thinking slower, and he's not contributing as much. I think he can do it. He just doesn't want to.

HE: I think I get myself so lazy, I have a hard time doing things that I enjoy doing. It could be apathy.

SHE: His outward actions are, "I'll do it when I get ready to do it." But, we still do pretty much what we used to do. We travel a lot, play cards, and he bowls. We got him onto a bowling team a couple of years ago. He goes hunting with his cousin and some buddies. He likes living in the woods for a while, watching the birds. The only thing is, it's not good for his Parkinson's because he's just sitting in a blind waiting for the animals to show up, so it's not much body and brain stimulation. When he comes back home, his mind is like jelly. I talk to him and he doesn't respond. I call it "la-la land." He doesn't get back in the groove of home right away. He goes a week in October and a week in November, and does other day trips, weather permitting.

HE: The doctor has mentioned DBS surgery quite a few times to me. He said I'd be a good candidate for it. He's given me the CD to watch, explaining it. As far as he knows me, he says it'll control the tremors.

SHE: I think it's because he mentioned the tremors and the doctor said, "If you want to entertain the idea, I'll go along with it."

HE: But I look at that as being the last straw. My mind doesn't think about my condition too often, but when I do think about it, I tell myself it could be worse. Others keep themselves afloat. I can keep myself afloat.

SHE: I have to learn to live with improvising. For me, this disease is a lesson in patience. He can sit at the table for an hour eating. I can't sit that long. I can take a bath, curl my hair, make a dinner for tomorrow, and he's still eating. My biggest challenge is just taking it one day at a time and not worrying about what's ahead. By the same token, I want to be aware and realistic, not in denial, about what's really happening, so if there's something we need to take care of we can.

HE: If I recognize I feel overloaded or stressed, the first thing I do is make sure I've taking my meds. Sometimes I vary too much on the time I take them. It takes me a long time to feel better.

SHE: If we have family or company over, I look, and he's wandered off. He doesn't want to be where the crowd is. I'll say, "Come on. Join in." He's doing less and less engaging in conversation. He doesn't even engage with me very much, just a couple of questions, then he wanders off. He will go downstairs to his gun room where he has hunting gear and his hunting trophies. He has mounted pheasant, deer head, elk head, and antelope.

HE: I'm on medication for depression. I have been for quite a few years, even before Parkinson's.

SHE: I wonder about Alzheimer's. He participates in a drug trial, and they have done a lot of memory testing. He seemed to score pretty well.

He's always fought the battle of depression. He'll talk about doing things on one hand, and he doesn't do them on the other. He chooses not to. I love doing a lot of things. I love sewing. I got an embroidery machine. I like to crochet. I love crafts. Anything creative. I've done tole painting, ceramics, and porcelain dolls.

HE: Now she's into quilts.

SHE: I'm new into it and I want to design one for a Parkinson's donation.

HE: A support group gives me the feeling that I'm not alone in the world and that there are other people struggling with the same thing. It makes me feel I have another family to turn to if I need someone to talk to or be with.

SHE: A support group is good. The kids don't really understand, and the friends don't, because they're not walking down the same path. They may read about it, but they don't get the full understanding of what's going on and don't see it on a day-to-day basis.

My advice to others would be, "Go to a neurologist that specializes in Parkinson's." If we'd gone to one in the beginning, we would have had the right diagnosis in the beginning. Join a support group because you learn about Parkinson's. We have speakers, exercises, things that give us hope, and ideas of what we can be doing.

HE: I feel I'm very lucky to be where I am, and I'm trying to enjoy everything I can. We've being going camping for 43 years. We've been to all 50 states.

SHE: I drive. We're going back to Colorado for two weeks. He's very good about travelling,

HE: I think, in a sense, whether it's my human nature, or Parkinson's, I've been excluding myself, or pulling myself away. It's like having a bubble over the top of me, not participating in conversation or thinking of fun things to do. It's hard to keep the mindset open. I don't want to admit to myself that I'm isolating myself.

SHE: He's always been like that. He didn't contribute much with friends.

HE: I think I've pulled back even more. I try to put more fun in life with my kids and grandkids. I try to joke and get them laughing and look at the fun side instead of the serious side. I think there are days I get up and tell myself that there's nothing wrong. I don't have a disease of any sort. But, when I take my pills, I realize there's something that I have to combat. You hear so much about different diseases, and the progress they're making, but they have no cure yet to get rid of PD. I'm wondering if I'm going to be around to see this happen.

I was a die maker, doing die repairs for an auto company. We've been married over 45 years. We met working at the same factory. We have a son and daughter, both married, and five grandchildren.

SHE: As a caregiver, I would say it takes a lot of patience and love and understanding. When I get overwhelmed, I take a break and go do something for a day.

HE: If I see I'm bugging her too much, I tell her to go out to lunch with the girls or go to her sewing class.

SHE: And I get a break when he goes hunting.

HE: We'll work it out together.

I'D RATHER PLAY BINGO

AGE: 72
DIAGNOSED: 10 years
Female Parkinson's Patient

I'm not used to having people in and talking to people.
I'm probably a loner.

The doctor said I don't blink as much as normal, which
affects my looks. To myself, I seem to be an old lady.
Just a couple of years ago I was so physical, and now
it's hard to do anything – to bend down and pick
something off the floor. I'd rather leave it there.

I was still working at a stamping and frame company, a
tier one company to the auto dealers. I did secretarial
work. When using the computer, the jjjjjjjjjjjjjj kept
showing up. Things like that. The company was going
to close anyway, so I didn't have any choice but to
retire. I retired eleven years ago.

I was going to physical therapy and I noticed my thumb
was going around on my index finger like crazy. The
physical therapist said, "You should see somebody
about that." I found a neurologist on my own. I just
remember that dark, dingy office in the basement of a
hospital.

I was probably about 62. I had been noticing things for
six months. I hadn't been concerned, but when the
neurologist said he suspected Parkinson's disease (PD),
I just started to cry. He sent me for a brain scan. He
said, "We better have one to be sure it's not something
else." The scan didn't show I had anything wrong, so
then he figured it was PD. I was upset, of course. But
he didn't give me any medicine or anything like that.
People asked me, "Why? There must be some
medication for it," meaning for the tremors.

I don't remember where I got the name of another
neurologist. Anyway, I went for a second opinion. She
said that I had it. They did a few physical tests, and

they noticed I didn't walk straight, my right arm just hung there, and the left arm swung naturally. My doctor put me on a mild dosage of medication.

I changed doctors because I had to wait two hours to see her and an hour to get in the room. I must have heard about a movement specialist through the support group. But, after a couple of years, I went back to her because she's closer. I'm on a Parkinson's medicine, and one for depression.

Nothing I was doing stopped right away. I was on the city Zoning Board of Appeals. I was babysitting and driving my granddaughter from school. When my hand would shake, she'd pat it and try to fix her Mimi.

I didn't think that Parkinson's would affect me much. I still did my own housework and yard work. It's really been the last year or two that it bothers me more. Now, with the changes, I am feeling afraid of the future.

I was angry that I couldn't do the things I wanted to. All I wanted was to be comfortable. I guess my biggest concern was that I would have to be taken care of by my family, that I would have things happen that I didn't want to have happen. I used to ride my bike around the neighborhood. I stopped about three years ago. With my lack of balance, I was afraid I was going to tip over.

I saw the support group listed in the paper. I went to learn more about what was going on. I got information from them and ordered the booklets and everything. I told my kids they might have to take care of me. I go off and on to the support group. I see people who have it so bad, so I don't go. I don't want to be like that.

My daughter wants me to have the brain operation. She probably wants to have me well again. She's seen me when I'm really slow and can't get up.

My neighbor had Parkinson's. She was bent over. The main impression I had was her at a church wedding being pushed down the aisle in a wheelchair, and her son helping her out of the wheelchair and taking her to the pew where the family of the bride sat. Then at the reception, I saw her husband feeding her. I thought "Oh gosh. That's me in the future. Who knows how long it will be?"

I get so tired, I drag my left foot sometimes. I have to remember to lift my leg up, like I'm marching in a parade. I have drooling at night.

I have freeze-up moments. I'm just standing there, and then I can't lift my feet. It's like heavy stones on the bottom of my legs. I just tell myself I have to move. I lift up my foot and I get going again.

I can't put on pantyhose or tights.

I think my voice is OK now, since they changed my medication, but my voice was really soft. It would just fade away like my handwriting does.

I've had urinary tract infections several times.

Sometimes, I have internal tremors. When I had my cold this winter, I must have had a fever and the tremors were going right to town.

Very seldom do I get a necklace or bracelet hooked up. It makes me mad that I can't wear them. I have to take them somewhere and have someone put them on me. My hands are getting so they feel kind of different. I can't hang onto stuff. If I hold a paper for a short time, my fingers just open up and it falls to the floor. My hands get quite stiff, and they don't stay on the computer keys right. Sometimes the A and the Z are mixed up.

I've been divorced about 27 years. I have two children, one locally, and four grandchildren. Both are married. I have a sister only 30 minutes away.

The kids would do something if I asked them to. The neighbors have been very nice, too. When I looked out yesterday on a snowy, icy day, my neighbor was using his snow blower on my walk and driveway. I live on a corner, so I have a long front and side area.

I've been very active in my garden and yard. I volunteer at the senior center, and I'm a churchgoer, and I like to play cards. Even after I retired from my job, I'd go back to play cards with the guys on their lunch hour. I still volunteer for the gift shop at the senior center. As long as I can handle money and the cash register, I'm OK. I still did some yard work this year. I now walk with a cane. My balance is off sometimes. I've fallen. I started falling last year. It's like you don't know you're going to do it. It's like there's a void or something. I can't stop myself. After falling a few times, my doctor wanted me to use a cane or a walker.

I don't feel too bad right now. I take some vitamins, but a lot of times I just feel like I have no strength or I'm just too darned tired. I miss out on things because I'm afraid to fly anywhere, worrying, "What if I don't feel good?" I get so weak, I'd be a bother to everybody. It's not a disease where people can see there's something wrong with you, so they don't think there is anything wrong with you.

My friends are more sympathetic. They know that something is wrong with me and that they have to help me out. One friend will drive me back and forth to my mother's and sister's, a 30 mile drive. Every week, I go up to see my mother. She's almost 95 years old.

I go to the movies. I like to read. I have friends I can call and talk to. I like to shop. I play Bingo every week at nearby senior centers, and I like to go three or four times a year on their casino trips. The medicine might be affecting my desire to gamble, but I keep it under control. I think if I lived near a casino, it would be hard for me, but I don't drive to the casino myself. I could go back and play five scratch-offs a day.

I'm proud that I can manage the computer enough to publish a four page listing of euchre games in the area, sponsored by a children's group. I take care of my finances responsibly.

My hands don't work like they used to. I've been to therapy for them. They're stiff, but also weaker. Therapy helps. I use the computer, but my left hand is dropping off and it's harder to do. I've got a machine I can ride for exercise, but don't. Every time I think of going back to exercise class at the senior center, I think, "ugh."

I had depression before, and it's about the same and that's with a low dosage of anti-depressant. Emotionally, I could cry easily, but taking my anti-depressant helps. I try not to take it sometimes, but it's better to stay on it, because I get shaky and can't handle everything. This way, I feel like I'm on an even keel.

I'm always losing my train of thought and I can't think of what I wanted to say.

I had carbon monoxide poisoning in 1960 from an old convertible that had plastic windows. Travelling across the state, I crawled back and wiped off the back windows. I crawled back up front and passed out, because of the fumes from the highway. I just read somewhere that they thought carbon monoxide may cause PD – as well as the fertilizers and insect repellants used around the house.

My advice to others with symptoms would be to see a good doctor. Who is a good doctor? Mine is always late. Be aware of, and certainly go to the support groups. Read all you can about PD. Make your house safe so you won't stumble and fall. I find that's happening to me more often. You can certainly take care of yourself by interfacing with others, and having a good doctor. I took the BIG and LOUD (LSVT) programs. They helped because my voice doesn't sound weak now. But it's so easy to get out of the habit of doing the exercises.

Now I feel like I'm OK alone. I've lived alone for over 20 years. There are so many people out there that are so much worse off than I am – both mentally, physically, and monetarily.

What has helped me the most is probably the support group and the leader, although I'm more a loner and don't go to the monthly breakfast. But if anything conflicts with Bingo, I'd rather play Bingo.

Something positive, I have a handicap sticker.

I'VE GOT A PROBLEM AND IT'S NOT IN MY HEAD

AGE: 73
DIAGNOSED: 12 years
Male Parkinson's Patient

I've aged. I don't look nearly as healthy as I used to. My body has taken a real beating in the last two to three years.

They had trouble diagnosing me. It started about 12 years ago with digestive problems.

I went to emergency one night. I had symptoms of a heart attack so I called my son. The doctor said, "I'm glad you came in." They put me in their cardio section. The doctor said, "It is good news. There's nothing wrong with your heart. But, you've got a digestion problem." I mentioned it to my family doctor. He said, "You better have someone take a look at you. You have gallstones. I recommend gall bladder surgery." It didn't help me any. I noticed certain foods were hard to digest. I continued to have digestion problems.

My primary doctor sent me to a gastroenterologist, who put me through every kind of test they could give me – colonoscopy, and exploratory upper and lower GI. "I couldn't find anything wrong. The pancreas looked OK," he said.

I told him, "I've got a problem. You can see I'm losing weight like crazy." He implied that there was something wrong with my head, that I was anorexic, and wanted to be thin. He said there was nothing else he could do.

The previous doctor's nurse, who had overheard the conversation, said, "Mr. H., I think you might want to go to the University of Michigan (U of M) doctor in the gastroenterology department. In the past, we've had people go there and meet with success."

I went to U of M – to a research doctor. I described my problem. "Well, Mr. H., I don't know if I can cure you, but I'll find out what's wrong with you." I said, "That's great." He used all the information accumulated from my past tests, asked for another test, and he did a lot of research. He called me a month later. "I know what's wrong with you. That's the good news. The bad news is I don't know how to cure you." I said, "What's wrong?" He said, "You have pancreatitis. It's not a physical problem. You're OK physically. It's a neurological problem. Your brain is not sending the message to the pancreas. The pancreas is supposed to create the digestive enzymes to digest your food." He had a stack of stuff from his research. "I think you have Parkinson's disease (PD). There are a small number of people with PD who are experiencing this problem." He also noticed from the reports that the only thing that was abnormal was an elongated bowel. That's the key. People with Parkinson's tend to have that elongated lower bowel because the muscles in the intestines don't work properly. It doesn't move the food along, so it tends to pile up over time and back up, which stretches or distorts the lower bowel.

Finally, after two years, I was happy to know that someone understood the problem. I'd heard of PD, but it was just a word. I didn't understand it. When I left his office, I had learned more about Parkinson's and the digestive system than from the previous specialist.

At that time, I had no other PD symptoms. The U of M gastroenterologist sent me to a neurologist and sent all my information to him. He did some tests, such as hitting me with a hammer, watching me walk, and pushing me to see if I'd fall over. I didn't have all the symptoms of classic PD. The second time I went back, he said, "You've got PD." I said, "I believe you, because the doctor at U of M is pretty intelligent."

At a family get together at Christmas, a friend said, "You know, your hand is shaking. You ought to go to the doctor." I told him, "I've already been." I didn't want to say it was Parkinson's. I don't like to admit I have PD to people because they treat you differently. They don't know anything about it. They don't know if you're carrying some kind of germ or virus. The rest of the family gasped, and kind of treated me different right away. Almost like, "stay away from me." They just didn't know, and thought it was kind of a hideous thing – that someone would lose control of their arms and legs – but all I had was a little tremor.

I kept going to the neurologist every month. I asked, "My God, what will we do for this?" He said, "We've got all kinds of meds to keep it under control." He started me out with medication given to people who have the flu, because they discovered it helps people with neurological problems. After about a month, I said, "This isn't helping me." All this time, I still couldn't digest food. So, he tried other things, and a combination of things. None of them really helped. The side effects were worse – diarrhea, nausea, insomnia, hallucinations, rather bad dreams, and nightmares.

Then I joined the local PD support group. I saw it listed in our local paper. That was about seven years ago. I went to the meeting and discovered I could get a lot of information. I started reading everything I could. The doctor knew the drugs being used for PD, but they weren't doing any good, and I was getting worse. I couldn't eat at all, and the tremors were getting worse. It was little things. The muscles were tightening up during the night.

I used to cross country ski 20 miles a day. I knew what it felt like to be in really good shape because I'd been that way most of my life. But, I knew something was going on, and I knew it wasn't old age, either. I used to get crazy pains. They'd come and go. I couldn't bend my thumb. I couldn't use a can opener. In the meantime, I went to a PD support group seminar and they brought different people in to speak. One night they had a neurologist who was a movement specialist, specializing in PD. Everyone seemed to think that he was the doctor to see. I asked him questions about things I had read. A woman mentioned she couldn't eat protein with her meds. I told him I couldn't either. He said, "No, that's not true," but he was wrong.

I didn't do anything for another six months. Then another specialist in neurology came to our support group and talked. She did a nice job and she was very personable. She listened. I was so tired of doctors that didn't listen. So, I went to see her. She is a movement disorder specialist. She tests your movement progress and does the other routine tests.

I'd always been a really active person. I skied at a lot of places around the world. It was my passion. When I'd fall and lose my balance, I used to rationalize it and say, "I must have crossed my skis." But, sometimes I'd fall standing in line to get a lift. I gradually phased out of skiing, and this year I quit altogether. I knew it was coming. I was prepared for it.

The hardest thing to cope with is the rigid schedule I have to stick to for my pill-taking. I have to be very careful because I still have intestinal problems. I have to take my medication on an empty stomach and keep proteins under control, otherwise I don't feel good. I get tired, and my vision begins to blur.

I feel my past heart problems were caused by bad diet. I ate poorly to keep from being hungry. I had four bypasses last August because of blocked arteries. I was in the hospital for three months during which time I got pneumonia, and then a MRSA infection. I was in rehab for three weeks. The hardest thing about this is the eating and the meds. I didn't fit in with their meal plan. I feel better when I can eat properly. I don't know how to solve the problem, and no one else does either. The medicine has to get in the small intestines before it is absorbed.

I'm on medication, but the problem is the effectiveness. The "on" time has become shorter and shorter. I used to take one pill every six hours. Now I'm taking 1 1/4 pills every two hours. Starting last week my doctor decided it might be a good idea to add another medicine in addition to my PD med to extend its effectiveness in my bloodstream and brain.

I discovered I was having trouble writing. It got so small, I couldn't even read it. That's when I gave up full time teaching, at age 55. I was teaching math part time at the college at the time of my tremor onset. I have a master's degree in mathematics.

I'm getting to be more of a recluse. My sphere of friends is shrinking. I divorced a year after I retired, and that's when I got PD. I used to be more gregarious. My life used to be based on relationships. It's not that way anymore. I go on a trip by myself. I went to Europe, Alaska, and Hawaii. I used to go skiing in Colorado and Nevada. I had a lot of ski friends. I can't participate in the sport and I don't fit in there anymore. I spend a lot of time at the library and I enjoy reading now. Before, I was too busy with people and never had time to go to the library.

I have a problem with walking. My big toe has an artificial joint and it's never been right. I don't know if it has anything to do with PD. It's from an injury 30 years ago. I walk kind of flat footed because I don't have an equal gait, and it throws my hip off. Once in a while, my legs seem stiff, but it goes away when I start moving. I went to an exercise class three times a week, but I couldn't keep up with the schedule. Some days I didn't feel good. I really couldn't perform because of fatigue and weakness. So, I set up a home gym that I can use when I feel strong enough.

Once in a while, I get a hoarse voice.

I didn't have problems falling until last week. I passed out and fell in my kitchen. It was an instant thing, and I came right back. It was the craziest thing. My son happened to be right next to me. I twirled around to get something, and I just went out. The cardiologist thinks it was low blood pressure.

I think my eye problems are related to PD. When I take my meds, the fogginess and out-of-focus vision will clear up within a half hour. My eyes water fairly easily.

I take medication all through the night, every two hours. I've never been in a state where I am not medicated. If I didn't take my meds throughout the night, I might not be able to get out of bed. As long as I keep my strict schedule with my meds, I'm OK.

My right arm doesn't swing nearly as much as my left. I have problems with my right shoulder. I used to sleep on my right side. I don't do that anymore. It hurts.

Sometimes I feel like I'm shaking inside, but nobody can see it.

I asked my doctor, "What happens when my medications don't work anymore? I've tried them all." She said, "We'll do DBS surgery." "I don't see where that will really help me that much," I said. "Seems to me it would be for people with movement disorders. If I don't have that problem, what good would it do?" Even though we talked to the surgeon at the hospital, I really don't want to do DBS. I did look into stem cell. I was close to going to China. I read more about it and saw some specials on TV about the scams out there. You really have to be very careful. It's illegal in the states and there's no guarantee. 1) You could get better, 2) You could get worse, or 3) You could die.

I don't have a very good sense of taste. I lost that, pretty much. Same with sense of smell. I've got a good appetite now, and I force myself to eat the proper things. I'm conscious of calories so I won't lose weight, but I still can't gain. My body burns up calories.

I get tired easy. Lately, I eat most of my protein at dinner, my last meal. Once I do, I can't do anything for the rest of the day. I just sit down and I'm knocked out.

I have one son who lives nearby. He's there if I need him, but we don't mention it much. He doesn't know much about the problem, but he probably knows more than he lets on. I have a granddaughter; they're healthy and very social. I'm a drag.

I am fearful about my situation, in a way. I was coming down a hill at 50 miles an hour, skiing, not long ago, and until now, felt that I could always figure out a way to get over every problem.

Since I'm by myself, I think about where I'm going to go, or what's going to happen to me. Lately, at times, I have depression. I usually find something to do, and it goes away. I worry about my memory, too, but it comes back to me eventually. I've got a new hobby building model railroads. I used to build them as a kid. It keeps me busy and I don't have to be real mobile.

I've done things I wanted to do and enjoyed my life. I can sit back and reflect on interesting wilderness trips I took out west, and different train rides I went on throughout the U.S. – places I enjoyed researching before I went.

I would say, if you have to go to a hospital for an operation, go somewhere that has knowledge of PD and the meds. They may not know about the effects of your medications.

My advice would be to get involved as much as you can with clinical research. Read all the data you can.

I feel like I would be hypocritical if I went to church and requested God to help now that I need help. I haven't been to church in years. I was a choirboy when I was a kid. I sang at Henry Ford's funeral in a big cathedral, St. Paul's Cathedral, on Woodward Avenue.

IT'S NOT A SHARP CUT-OFF OF YOUR LIFE

AGE: 77
DIAGNOSED: 12 YEARS
Male Parkinson's Patient

You have to be patient with me. I talk so softly, others have a problem hearing me. And, my speech is halting, too. In hindsight, I was probably already talking fairly quietly when I started noticing my shakiness. I noticed it particularly when holding a hymnal in church. The pages would flutter.

My brother had Parkinson's disease (PD). Since we are very similar in physical traits and appearance, I almost anticipated it, and I was not surprised when I was diagnosed. My brother and I are so much alike that, when my kids were younger, they ran up to him calling him "daddy." He was quite a bit older than I am – eight years older. By the time I had symptoms, I knew about his. At first, he denied he had Parkinson's, and so did his wife. We rarely got together, so I hadn't seen him to notice how he was doing until he was almost bedridden. I had heard that he had been restricted from driving. He had always carried a pocket knife and that was taken away. I don't know why. It might have been his wife's apprehension. He also wore more pajama-type clothing, without a belt.

I was diagnosed around age 65. By that time, I knew what the prospects were and what the sequence of events would be. However, I realized it might be a different time scale for me. It was a matter of accepting, "What will be, will be."

One of the earliest signs for me, which we didn't realize was significant, was the loss of the sense of smell. Also, I experienced the loss of my fine motor movements. I had a hard time brushing my teeth. Now I brush two-handed. I use my left hand to help control my right. Early on, my handwriting became small and less legible. My voice was raspy and harsh. I have difficulty stating something loud enough to be heard. I have taken the LOUD program. I have to remember that my voice quality isn't there, and I have to deliberately use the tools I've learned in order to be heard.

Those changes weren't affecting my life that much. I don't remember that there was anything specific I couldn't do. But, I was probably beginning to be a little slower, or a little more cautious, and fearful about stumbling.

Eventually, I asked my primary doctor for a reference to see a neurologist. I'm sure I didn't think it was Parkinson's disease at first. But as soon I noticed the tremors, and knowing about my brother, I thought, "The sooner I can get treatment, the better."

The neurologist diagnosed PD because of lack of my arm swinging when I walked, tremors, although very mild, and masking. I thought my lack of facial expression was due to the fact that I had adapted a stoic demeanor, a poker face, in order to testify in court as a corporate representative.

I wasn't too concerned about the changes taking place because I thought it would be a long time before I would progress to the stage that would incapacitate me. I was thinking, "I do have Parkinson's, and I'm not surprised that I do, but I'll have quite a few long years before extreme disability."

Another thing I noticed was a tendency to lightheadedness. At the time, I was flying quite a bit. On one trip, I had to really concentrate when getting off the airplane and slow down and stand for awhile. Getting up out of a chair at a restaurant, I would black out for seconds by the time I got to the door. My blood pressure would drop so quickly that I'd pass out. I just attributed it to the fact I'd been sitting down a long time. It turned out to be orthostatic hypotension. I've eliminated my blood pressure medicine because of the lightheadedness. I wear compression hose for low blood pressure.

We heard about a Parkinson's support group from someone I met at the local senior center. We found that in this support group there are about seven men with Parkinson's who are engineers. That's what I was trained to be.

While attending the local support group, I would hear people talking about a certain medication they were taking. So, I started asking my doctor about it. My doctor wasn't a movement disorder specialist. We learned of a doctor who was, and when he spoke at one of the first support groups we attended, I switched to him as my doctor.

I feel the same as ever. However, I'm a little more lethargic. I have more trouble with buttons. I don't think I've been depressed. I've had several things that are difficult to accept, such as managing personal decisions and documents. I used to just step up and do those things. Now it's more anxiety-producing, so I procrastinate. I know I'm not participating socially when I could. I feel like I don't participate because I'd have to butt in. So, I feel left out socially sometimes. It feels lonely.

I've always been a pretty heavy reader. I read technical things. I do fix-it jobs around the house and I like repairing electrical things. I used to enjoy gardening. I like using the computer to communicate with friends, looking on YouTube, and reading or sending about 100 emails a day.

The hardest thing to cope with is feeling isolated because of memory difficulty, not being able to think of the right word. I don't know if it's a senior moment. Circulating with other people helps, but it still feels bad not to know the name of someone I was talking to yesterday. I try to rationalize that others my age have the same problem.

I was born on a farm in Northern Wisconsin. My dad had been recruited during World War II by recruiters who traveled the farm country to find out who might be interested in coming to Detroit to work in the factories. He was a pretty good mechanic. He hauled us down to Michigan in a Ford pulling a homemade trailer behind.

I'm one of ten children. I realized, to get anywhere, I'd have to get a college education. We all earned our own way and put ourselves through college. I earned my way through General Motors Institute's Co-Op, doing alternate months of work and school. G.M.I. was primarily for engineering professions. So that's what I was trained to be. I took "30 and out" and retired. After I retired, I started my own consulting company, with which my wife helped.

We married after having lived almost next door to one another since grade school. Our immediate family is our two boys, one living in Colorado, the other nearby.

When they describe someone coming out of their shell, that's me. The Parkinson's support group has done that for me. They're all so friendly. Parkinson's is not a sharp cut off of your life. You don't have to be confined. You can associate with other people, particularly those who can understand the disease. Parkinson's is not something you brag about, but it's not something you have to whine about, either.

[See his spouse's story on the following pages.]

WE'VE BEEN DOING OK

Female Spouse

Here I'm supposed to be the caregiver for him, and I feel like he's taking care of me. I was in the hospital twice so far this year. He has been making sure I have what I need. I'm very fortunate that his Parkinson's is not that bad. He is slow, but that doesn't keep him from doing things.

People may not think of him as having Parkinson's, because not that many people know about Parkinson's. They know something's wrong with him, but they think he has had a stroke. I'm thinking of when we're in a restaurant. If he orders something, he's slower and he speaks softly. If they can't hear him, they won't ask him to repeat it, but they'll look at me for help to understand what he said. I feel sorry because I don't want people to misinterpret, and I don't want to be ashamed of him.

My family tends to interrupt a lot. We'll be sitting around talking – six or eight people. He's a little slower in getting started to say something, and by the time he gets it out, the group has gone on to another topic. So, I've told him to interrupt, but he's never been a loud, aggressive person. He is quiet and reticent in public.

Early on, I noticed he had the masking, an expressionless face. I can't tell you exactly when. It was one of the earlier symptoms. He also had a little stooping and hunched shoulders. It's kind of funny, because we can't remember how long it's been since he's been diagnosed. I think it's been at least ten years. What makes me feel good is, although I notice his tremors have increased in the last year, he doesn't seem to be getting worse, or more handicapped. The condition is not keeping him from doing anything. He's just primarily slower in accomplishing things, slower in dressing.

He takes care of his meds himself. I'm not involved in that.

I don't know that I had a difficult time accepting his diagnosis. His brother had Parkinson's. I do wish things were different for him, but I think the thing that makes him most angry is when I try to protect him from doing things, like his climbing on a ladder and changing a light bulb. He feels I should be more encouraging. But, even the doctor has said to him, "I don't want you to crack your head open." He has fallen a few times. I'm more concerned that he might get an injury that will lay him up more than the Parkinson's does. I say, "Don't climb the ladder. Wait for our son."

He has a mild temperament. He comes from a family of ten children. His whole family is calm, not loud, not angry, but soft-spoken. I can't remember any of them raising their voice or yelling at anyone ever.

The hardest thing for me to adjust to is his slowness, and having to wait for him. Like, if we're getting ready to go somewhere, I can get my coat on and he's still putting his shoes on. I have to remember that I don't have to start getting ready as early as he does. But now, he's doing for me, because I'm wearing a back brace. So how can I be angry when he's helping me now put my coat on, and he's caring for me, more than I'm caring for him?

Even so, he will say sometimes I hover too much. I don't think I do, because I think I'm protecting him. I think our doctor would agree with me. For instance, I close the door to the downstairs to keep him from going down. His computer is downstairs in the basement and he likes it down there so he can spread his stuff out. His blood pressure was dropping when he'd get up too quickly after sitting so long. He got lightheaded coming up the basement stairs. He had a little bit of an issue passing out.

Otherwise, anything he wants to do, I think he's pretty much doing. He's going to a personal trainer now. He goes to the Computer Club at the senior center. He's reading or working on the computer most of the day. He'll be putzing in the garden in the summertime. He works on his son's lawnmower or fixes anything mechanical when needed.

After 30 years with GM, he took an early retirement. After retirement, he went into business for himself. We worked together. I did the office work. He is a man with a good reputation; smart and well respected in the business world. I don't want anything to diminish that.

I don't do enough about my own well-being. I'm not active enough, but my back restricts me – he doesn't. I like sewing, quilting, needlework, and crocheting.

We get our emotional support from each other, and we have a certain amount of faith. We've had a very good marriage. No anger or shouting. That just doesn't happen.

There should be more awareness of Parkinson's disease because people don't know enough about it. I think the support groups are important, because if you're having a problem, you can find out how someone else handled it. One of the things about the support group, we see people at all stages, and have empathy for them and want to share. We have three events a month: the monthly Wednesday night informative meeting, the monthly caregivers support group, and the monthly Monday morning breakfast. We get together socially for special events, too. We've probably become more social and we have enlarged our circle of friends through the Parkinson's disease support group.

My words of encouragement are, just count your blessings. If you look around you, there's always someone having a more difficult time than you.

I think we're blessed that, for say ten years, we've been doing OK.

A FAMILY AFFAIR

AGE: 77
DIAGNOSED: 14 years
SHE: Parkinson's Patient
WE: Son and Daughter-in-law of Female Patient

Until this last year, progression of mom's Parkinson's disease (PD) had been very slow. In the last year, however, she's been declining.

That's probably because she fell last autumn. She'd been living with us for four years. It was a really nice day. She had been sitting on the front porch. She wanted to feel useful, so she got up to rake a few leaves. She gets a bee in her bonnet, and she wants to finish something she shouldn't have started. She gets dizzy and her body gets too tired and she shuts down. She looked like she had been in a prizefight, with bruises and cuts and broken toes and teeth.

She's never fully recovered since then. She was in the hospital for three weeks when she fell. Then she went back in for a couple of days with an inflamed colon. Then a couple of months later, she went back with a bowel obstruction. When she went in for her bowel obstruction, they put a colostomy bag on. At that time they said, "If recovery goes well, in six or eight weeks, we'll reverse the surgery." It didn't happen that fast because she was having problems with hallucinations, dehydration, weakness, and several urinary tract infections. She can't be alone right now, as she has fallen a few times.

Since autumn, she hasn't been home for any length of time. She's been in and out of two hospitals, two rehab centers, and right now is in assisted living. She is scheduled to go back into the hospital in two weeks to reverse the colostomy.

During all this, it's like she has no more will. Our biggest concern is that she's giving up and not even trying. We don't want to see her in the nursing home for the rest of her life.

During her hospital stay, they thought she might have dementia because of the way she acted while there. We said, "No, we don't think so. This is not typically the way she behaves." They might have just assumed that dementia was the next step because she has PD. They tried to cut back her medicine because of hallucinations, but she became too agitated. She's been using her wheelchair, and not her walker. She's been having leg cramps. Just this week, the neurologist re-upped her meds. Within hours, once she was back up to her regular dosage, we saw an improvement in her fatigue, lethargy, and leg cramping. It's only been a couple of days, so we don't know yet if she'll get hallucinations again.

Mom was diagnosed with Parkinson's disease 14 years ago, at age 63. I don't know how long she had the symptoms before she was diagnosed. At the time, we really didn't know that much about Parkinson's. Dad was still alive, and we thought, "OK, we'll deal with it." Her writing and shaking were the first signs. Her writing got smaller. Dad was partially retired and they went to a neurologist and got a firm diagnosis, and then she started on the Parkinson's medication. What I don't remember is how she reacted to the diagnosis. She expected my dad to be around to take care of her. They were married for 47 years and there are five of us children, 17 grandchildren, and 9 great grandchildren. After he died, 13 years ago, she acted like, "I'm disabled. I have this disease."

I would say mom has had depression, probably ever since dad's death. Her depression is probably a combination of the Parkinson's and her grief. Her kids and her grandkids have always been around.

She always acted kind of helpless, not wanting to take any initiative, not wanting to do things. She worried about things. We've pushed her to do things. She'd say, "I can't, because I have PD. I can't because I'm disabled." It became an excuse for her. The challenge is to let her know we love her and we're not being mean to her.

She stopped driving about five years ago. She didn't feel comfortable behind the wheel anymore. We took her up to the senior center where she volunteered, and she did exercises and physical therapy. We tried to show her that there are people there looking for friendships, too. She played Domino's once a month and she's been a Red Hat lady with her church group.

After she sold her house, she went into an independent living place. It cost a lot of money, and she didn't use the facilities she was paying for. We didn't feel she needed assisted living at that time.

Her daughters were already emotionally exhausted from managing her constant phone calls and her negative attitude. We all tried to encourage and bolster her up. They had been dealing with her neediness for eight years.

She moved in with us. At first, it was just, "There's someone else in the house with us. Pick up your stuff so grandma doesn't trip on it." Then she started telling the kids what to do. That's when we had to explain appropriate boundaries.

The first weekend she moved in, she waited until we were home and asked us to fix her a cup of tea. She was perfectly capable of taking care of herself. It was just her loneliness. She wanted companionship. The first year it was a constant battle to get her to get out and go to the senior center. We would drive her, but she'd say, "I'm woozy. I can't do this." We didn't know if she was trying to manipulate us, since her symptoms would come and go.

(Son) Denial is the way I cope. I'm not a caregiver. She just lives with us. It's hard for me to separate her personality from her physical problems. We don't know how to measure her behavior. When she came to live with us, our objectives were very clear. We set the boundaries, "We're not taking care of you. You're living with us." My wife had to deal with her the first year on a day-to-day basis. Then, she went to work. It gave her more autonomy and mom more breathing room.

(Daughter-in-law) It affected me the most. I had to turn my world upside down that first year to accommodate mom. I would make sure she had meals. But, if I went out, I felt like, "I have to get home because I've got to get mom taken care of." She'd follow me and ask, "How long are you going to be gone? When are you going to be home?"

Only if you know the symptoms of Parkinson's would you notice mom's facial masking. We took her to a play a year ago. The neighbor thought mom hadn't enjoyed the play because of her blank facial expression. She looked like she was mad or not enjoying herself. I had to explain, "Oh no. She enjoyed it. She expressed verbally she did. That's just her Parkinson's."

Her voice has always been a problem. It has always been hard to hear her and understand her. She would say something to the kids and they wouldn't respond because they couldn't hear her. She felt they were ignoring her.

Her walking has been a problem. Before she started using the walker, she shuffled, and if she tried to take longer steps, she'd say, "I can't." She does little short stumbling steps. If she would stop and start up again, her steps would be more normal. The walker helped, as it was a visual cue that, "Now I have something to walk to." There's a new walker out with a laser that puts out a red line as a visual cue to help you walk to it.

We noticed her rigidity when she was in the hospital this last time. Before that, she had flexibility and could still climb the stairs.

When at home, she sat in the chair and leaned way over to one side, and just hung there. We'd say, "Mom, can you sit up straight?" She complained that her back hurt. "Mom! Posture. You've got to work on your posture."

She's had severe leg cramps. We found a remedy, a proven old Amish formula; apple cider vinegar, ginger, and garlic. She says it works.

Mom had cataract surgery. At one point, they diagnosed her with macular degeneration. Another doctor said, "No, you don't have it." That was years ago. The last time she was at the eye doctor they said, "Well, you might have it." She complains that things look wavy, but when she has eye checks, they don't find anything. It comes and goes. She felt there were tremors in her eyes. The eye doctors keep telling us it has nothing to do with the PD.

She always carried a hankie or tissue for a drippy nose.

She would sometimes say, "I need my meds because I'm tremoring on the inside." We experienced her full body tremors when she was shaking all over because of anxiety. Her anxiety caused her blood pressure to be super high; 210 over 180. It eventually came down and the tremor attack went away.

To make it easier for her to dress, most of her clothes are pull-on pants and over the head tops. Her shoes are mostly slip-ons. She solved other grooming problems by going to the beauty parlor once a week to have her hair washed and set.

Her appetite has been very poor. She would eat more when I sat with her than if she ate alone. She does love her sweets, though.

Occasionally we cut her meat for her, but for the most part, we'd encourage her to try.

We assume mom has had vivid dreams because we've heard her screaming very loud. We have our door closed, and are on the other end of the house. She says she doesn't remember them.

We got her to go to grief counseling about two years after dad died. She was still living in their house. We finally convinced her to take something for depression. She seemed happier, but when she was on an antidepressant, she said she had a lot of sexual urges. She was more aggressive around males. She stopped taking the meds because she didn't want to feel or act like that.

She had piano lessons as a child. She always played for children's church when she was a Sunday school teacher. Her faith, since childhood, has carried her through to this day.

Even when she was leaving the hospital recently, and going to the first rehab place, she was somewhat confused, but she was quoting Bible verses.

Her belief is that God is in control. God is sovereign. She knows she's not supposed to be anxious, but she still is. She would be very proud of her legacy in that her kids and grandkids embrace her Christian faith.

APPRECIATE TODAY – TOMORROW WILL CHANGE

AGE: 84
DIAGNOSED: 14 years
Male Parkinson's Patient

My neurologist said he can tell if a person has Parkinson's by looking at them. If people know what to look for, they may notice I have Parkinson's because of a lack of expression in my face, and the fact that I stoop from the waist.

Most of the time, I don't think about the Parkinson's, but if I go to stand up and walk to the refrigerator, I make sure I have my walker. I still have to watch my balance and be careful about where and how I'm walking. I fall if I'm not paying attention.

I have a hard time standing up straight. I tend to fall backwards when I lose my balance. In fact, the first thing I noticed was that I would fall backwards when I was in the bathroom shaving.

That was 14 years ago. I mentioned it to my internist when I went for a checkup. He didn't say anything then, but a time or two later, he noticed I didn't have a swing in my arms when I walked. He set up an appointment for me to go to a neurologist who went through the little tests – checking the movement of my hands, my strength, and balance. The neurologist told me I had Parkinson's disease (PD).

He prescribed a couple of meds. I went to him every three months, and one time he got upset with me when I was a week late. I wondered if he was interested in me or something else. It was about that time that I started going over to the Parkinson's support group and decided to change to a movement specialist, even though it was a lot further to go. He put me on just one pill, where the other doctor had me on several. I got the same results. Information I had gotten about PD seemed to always mention medications being "on" or "off." If I feel like I'm "on," I can walk with a better, smoother step. Most of the time, I take accentuated, real short steps, like a shuffle.

I freeze anytime I go through a doorway or pass somebody. In our condo association, three of us ride together to a men's breakfast. One of them will stop and hold the door. If I'm not real careful going through the doorway, I stop on a dime and freeze. I could have gone through that doorway 1000 times in the past, but I still have the same freezing, and it gives me a helpless feeling because I have no control over it. Someone can be right behind me, but I still can't move and get out of the way. I just have to shuffle and pull myself through with the walker.

I use a special walker all the time – one that was supposed to be designed for PD patients.

I was recently widowed after 27 years of marriage and I live alone. It's tough when you have to depend on yourself. Back pain is the result of an injury I suffered years ago. I try to fix a meal, or make a sandwich for lunch, but when I'm on my feet, my back starts aching and I have a hard time. I get to the point I feel like I can't move. The doctor said old age could cause some of my problems.

I have drooling during the day. If I'm bending over to pick up something, drool flows out of my mouth.

I've noticed a lot of difference in my writing. I used to be an automotive designer and could write instructions on drawings in a straight line with letters all the same size. Now my writing is smaller and it is getting harder to read.

I have a feeling I'm losing my voice. I feel that I'm speaking at a normal volume, the volume that I always spoke, but people are asking me to repeat things. When I'm in a restaurant ordering a meal, the waitress will ask me to repeat the order again.

I can't distinguish what it is about my speech. I guess there is a hesitation, because I'll stop and think what I'm going to say before I speak. I'm more apt to be a listener now than a talker. I want to feel like I'm participating, but I'm not able to all the time. It's like I have a feeling that others don't want to hear what I have to say. I guess it makes me feel left out a little.

I'm having trouble seeing. I just recently stopped taking the newspaper because I had all the columns drifting back and forth looking like it was double-printed. I read in a book that PD will affect your eyesight. I told my eye doctor I was having trouble and I thought it was the PD. He didn't say anything. Sometimes even the printing across the bottom of the screen on television is not readable to me. It's been eight months since I've had new glasses. I went back in. They just adjusted the stems and thought it would help, but I got home and it didn't.

I have the most problems first thing in the morning, getting up on my feet and keeping my balance without falling backward. I have clothes nearby so I can get dressed without a lot of problems. That's the biggest part of the day sometimes, because it takes so long to get up, go to the bathroom, get my shoes on, and take my medication.

I have a young lady who comes in three times a week. She fixes meals for me. I don't eat as much as I used to. You can say I lost my appetite.

Occasionally, I exercise downstairs on the stationary bike, and I have some weights I use. I used to get up and work out for a half hour. I don't anymore. Either the weather conditions are not right or I put other things in front of it. Even like today, by the time I get moving around, a lot of time has gone by, and I find I'm tired out from just coping with the symptoms of my illness. I can't walk very far or very fast.

I've had a lot of problems with constipation. I have some powder to mix with a juice. That seems to help, but I'm at the point where I'm real conscious of it. If I'm going someplace or doing something, I don't want to get caught in a crowded place for obvious reasons.

I've noticed here just recently that if I go to lift my right arm to reach for something, I get some discomfort. I don't know if it's from PD, or if it's the way I lay in bed sleeping.

It's hard to tell when I lost my sense of smell. It's been a long time.

I used to play golf regularly. We went to Florida for a couple of months each winter, but it's been several years now since I've even been able to play golf. I gave my clubs to my son.

I'm stiff, and I need to be extra careful getting out of the car, even when I ride for only a little distance with the fellows in the subdivision. I haven't driven for over a year. The doctor said I shouldn't because I'm in stage three. It feels like hell – like I've lost part of my life and my freedom. When my wife was living, if she wanted to go to the market or shopping center, we'd jump in the car and go. Pretty soon, she was doing all the driving, which was alright with me. The last thing in the world I'd want would be to get into an accident and have someone injured. But, I felt like I could've kept driving. I didn't feel any weaker.

One of my biggest challenges is being patient enough to put up with not having any transportation. If I want to go someplace or do something, I have to wait until somebody comes along. People always say, "Just call and let me know," but that doesn't always go over big, either.

The concern I have about the future is not knowing what might happen, of losing control, and not being able to manage my affairs. I've already looked at a senior retirement community. I feel that once I leave my home, there'll be no coming back, no matter how much I like or dislike the place. I don't want to be a burden to someone, but I am partly now. Three of my four kids live fairly close by, and they come over and spend time with me. I've been fortunate that they have been really helpful.

The thing that makes me more aware of my condition is seeing a fellow with a power chair who comes to church nearly every Sunday. He lives in a nursing home nearby. I see him stand up out of his chair when he sings and I'm always concerned he's going to end up falling. He has Parkinson's. You can't hear him speak – he has no volume in his voice at all. His strength is practically non-existent, but he goes to church. After church, he uses the ramp and goes back to the nursing home. I guess I feel like if I ever get to that point there won't be much quality in life.

I think a support group is a lot like its name. It's a place people can get help and information about their disease that they may not get from a doctor; a place to help people cope with the Parkinson's symptoms and their condition. My father had Lou Gehrig's disease. He wasn't aware of any place he could go to get information or support. He more or less got upset with the doctors because he thought they could have done more.

It's hard to imagine how many things you have to cope with when you have a death in the family – my wife's death three months ago. My wife was a wonderful woman and she helped me the most. I put a load of responsibility on her, even though I tried to do things that were difficult for me to do because of my physical condition.

Even though my advice is to learn to accept what you have, I wonder what is coming next – things that I can't foresee that might change my style of living.

The hardest thing about the disease, and my condition, is coping with my lack of freedom. I try to keep active and handle every day as it comes. I guess the best thing out of all this, is, I've learned to appreciate what I have.

[Author's Note]

He appreciated his life before his death – three months after this interview.

BE YOUR OWN ADVOCATE

AGE: 71
DIAGNOSED: 15 years
HE: Parkinson's Patient
SHE: Spouse

SHE: "Why does grandpa look so mad?" That's the question our four granddaughters ask.

HE: I think it's because I have some masking and staring. I stoop and I shuffle. I have trouble walking. I use a walker, pretty much. In 1998, I was walking to the parking lot and noticed that I didn't swing my left arm. My left hand stayed in place and vibrated with tremors. I also had a problem washing my hair. I was age 56. I went to my primary doctor after that.

SHE: His primary doctor suspected he had Parkinson's disease (PD). He referred him to a neurologist who ran a few tests to rule out other things. We went to him every six months for a couple of years, before switching to a movement disorder specialist.

HE: I felt curious when I found out I had PD. It didn't seem so bad at first. It wasn't bothering me that much. I was director of electronics at General Dynamics. However, 12 years ago, Parkinson's was affecting my ability to do the job and I retired. I was around 60.

SHE: We didn't keep it from our two children. Our son is a doctor, so he's been with us all the way.

HE: My voice is quieter than it used to be. I'm very slow to talk. I don't write much anymore, because my writing is getting smaller and smaller.

SHE: He had shoulder problems at the very beginning. Going through doorways caused him to freeze up and is still a problem. It doesn't happen all the time. You just never know when it's going to happen. Also, I wondered about his nose dripping. It's an uncontrolled, sudden drip, like a drippy faucet, and it's always clear.

HE: I had trouble with my eyes. I couldn't read the newspaper. I had some special glasses made with prisms. I can read pretty well now. The ophthalmologist did a terrific job.

SHE: A couple of years ago, he told the doctor he was having double vision when he was driving. The doctor said, "You might want to try prism glasses." We didn't do anything about it at that time. When he went for an eye test, the test came out pretty good, but there was still something wrong. He got the prism glasses a couple of weeks ago. Now he reads the newspaper and can read from his Kindle.

HE: I get internal tremors and it's usually associated with some stressful situation. Sometimes it's the arm, sometimes it's the whole side. I would be shaking so that it would keep me from doing things with my hands, too. I've had vivid dreams and hallucinations, depending on the meds I've taken.

SHE: We've been going to the local support group about six years. I saw an article in the paper about one of the members who had Deep Brain Stimulation surgery (DBS).

HE: Then I had DBS surgery, and that didn't work out that good. I had the surgery last year because, well, I guess I qualified for it through my neurologist.

SHE: He had DBS surgery because the number one issue was dyskinesia (involuntary movements) in his upper body. The surgery did take care of that, but it's not a "cure all." Sometimes it can increase other symptoms. They'll tell you that up front. The freezing, they say, will never get better, nor will it help with balance. He feels that his balance got worse. I think we felt the benefits would outweigh the risk.

HE: That's the thing with DBS, it'll improve some things, but it sometimes makes things worse. You don't know ahead of time. Before DBS, I didn't have a problem with balance. Now, I fall often, several times a day. I don't drive.

SHE: After DBS, his mental state was disturbing. He was confused and suffered from memory loss. It could have been the meds still in his system. Or, as you get older, I guess the anesthesia might have caused it. He was supposed to be in the hospital just one night. He ended up in the hospital for five nights because of confusion, and wanting to get out of bed, which he was not allowed to do. After DBS, the doctor wanted him off certain meds because he was having vivid dreams.

After his DBS, we switched neurologists to get a second opinion. We changed because we were not happy. She was recommended to us, though she's not a movement specialist. So many times, I have come home from the doctor's office, frustrated and depressed because I didn't learn anything. With her, there is a rapport for me, and he likes her too. I've learned more from her than I did from our last doctor, who was more a researcher – not a people person. This new neurologist got the records from our hospital where the DBS surgery was done. She ordered a PET scan which showed dementia and Alzheimer's. We were confused that it showed up five months after the DBS surgery, whereas, before the DBS, he passed the written and oral tests, the standard testing required before doing DBS. He's taking meds now for memory loss.

I'm concerned about issues, such as falling. To me it's a big plus if I can keep him out of the hospital. I've seen others pick up infections in the hospital because their immune system was compromised as a Parkinson's patient. I just know that I don't want to go to the hospital unless we absolutely have to. He's more fragile, and I really feel like I have to work hard to keep him healthy.

HE: To go out we have to make sure everything is OK at the other end of the situation. I have to have time to go to the bathroom.

SHE: Leaving the house, you have to think about medicines you will need, water you will need to take with you, the availability of restrooms, and feelings of anxiety in social gatherings. As a care-partner, I share the stress. Our socializing is spread out now because he tires easily. Sometimes it's a good day, and sometimes it's a bad day. An outing one day might cause him to be extremely tired the next. Sometimes I think, "We shouldn't do this. It's too much for him to handle all at once." Another concern is wondering if his meds will be working that day.

HE: Now I'm more fearful of what's going to happen because I've seen two "fellow travelers" experience death by complications of Parkinson's. To cope, I'd say I turned to religion, but it's very hard to go to church, because I have to get everything set up at both ends.

SHE: It's very hard to get to church. He'll say, "I'll just lie down for five minutes. Wake me up." But, I won't. Sometimes we make it, sometimes we won't. I tell him, when he gets down on himself, "Look what you have to go through to get there." We have to really plan ahead, because he has to go to the bathroom, or because he'll get very tired.

HE: I watch sports. I can't get enough of MSU basketball. I went to MSU grad school for Wildlife Biology. I do spend time outside in the summer. I used to love to fish.

SHE: We met at work, an aerospace company. I was a secretary. My hobby is my husband right now. Before, it was gardening. We used to boat a lot, and I went fishing with him. The Parkinson's stopped us from boating. It was getting too risky with his balance problem, and the care and maintenance of a boat was getting overwhelming.

We used to cross-country ski. A group of around 20 people used to take trips planned by the nature center, with a guide. After he retired, we went to Puerto Rico,

Costa Rica, Mexico, Algonquin, Canada, and Isle Royale. Isle Royale is very wild, so we didn't camp. We don't travel anymore.

SHE: My outlook is to just get through this day and not dwell on things. Some days are better than others. Some people have it a lot worse than we do. And, we're fortunate we live close to our children, who are pretty attentive. The hardest thing is the fear of the future.

HE: I would advise others: "Don't get DBS."

SHE: We have a support group that meets monthly, a monthly breakfast, a caregivers meeting, a Christmas party, and a summer picnic. Another thing we do is the gala, an annual fundraiser.

HE: The support group is very important to us because it brings like-minded people together. It's important to have that kind of interaction. We meet people we never knew before, and they become our very good friends.

SHE: People who are not with him all the time don't understand. They may shy away because of fear of the unknown. They don't know what to say. That's why the support group is so nice – people can relate. We have a common bond with the others there.

HE: It provides information.

SHE: I think you have to be your own advocate. We try to read as much as we can about the disease. Also, if you're not happy with your doctor, then you should switch.

I FEEL A LOT, LOT BETTER WHEN I'M
LAUGHING

AGE: 76
DIAGNOSED: 15 years
SHE: Parkinson's Patient
HE: Spouse

SHE: Because I have masking, I consciously try to smile more and be more relaxed so I don't look like a ghost. When I get my nails done, they tell me to hold still.

I have a lot of different health problems. I have scoliosis, spinal stenosis, osteoporosis, and a degenerative disc, which gives me a bad tilt. I've had a tilt for a long time, as long as my husband can remember. I try to stand up straight, but I am getting pretty twisted. I know I'm only going to get worse. I go to a well-known spine doctor who wants to put rods in my spine. I don't want to go through that. I don't think it'll contribute to a better life at my age.

Fifteen years ago, I was in the middle of having my rotator cuff repaired and I had to have a primary doctor refer me before I could go into surgery. As I was checking out at the front desk, he was watching me walk, and he said, "Mrs. W., I think you have Parkinson's disease (PD). Your arm doesn't swing." He gave me some medication, but I concentrated more on my shoulder surgery and didn't do much about the Parkinson's diagnosis. I've since heard that with Parkinson's you could also have shoulder problems, and I wondered if it was related. Then I had back problems. I would crawl sometimes, the pain was so bad.

I would say I had PD even before I was diagnosed, but I didn't go to a neurologist for years. I had lost my sense of smell long before anyone thought of Parkinson's. My gait was bad. My whole family walks kind of funny, kind of tilted to the side. My husband just thought it was a family trait, but as years went on, I knew my gait was different. Just by feeling, I could tell. A few people suggested I go to a neurologist.

I went to a neurologist and she said I didn't have PD. Then I went to another neurologist. He thought I did. He started me off on some medication, but he didn't know about PD and I didn't either. Nothing seemed to work right, but I kept going the way I was going. My gait was off, I didn't have smell, but I didn't shake. We were just so busy with everything else in our life.

I went without meds for a long time. My primary doctor prescribed some eventually, but in the meantime, I got bit by a bug and was treated for six months for Lyme disease. I was on intravenous feeding for eight months. I tested positive for lupus, too. My neurologist called the specialist for Lyme disease a quack. No one wanted to talk about it or treat it. It's too controversial.

I had gone to a couple of other neurologists. Seven years ago, I went to a recommended neurologist who specializes in movement disorders.

I wish I knew then what I know now. I didn't know about all of the symptoms of PD and what the outlook might be. The doctor didn't tell me anything. I would have planned a little differently. We just went on doing what we were doing. I would have taken it easier. I might have travelled or had more fun. Instead, we built a 6000 square foot home on a lake. It took a couple of years to build. We moved so many times. We sold a home and rented a home until we built a home. It caused a lot of stress and conflict that we could have done without.

My brother has had Parkinson's for five or ten years. He keeps it pretty much to himself. He's a chiropractor. He'll be 75 next month. We were raised in the country. That's what I attribute it to. We used to have that tin sprayer that we used with bug spray to spray the house often because we had a lot of flies. I think he walks a lot different than me and has a lot more fatigue than I do.

HE: He has a major voice problem. I remember years ago, before I knew anything about Parkinson's, I would come home from a family get-together and say, "You know, I just don't like talking to your brother because I can't hear him." He couldn't get his voice out to talk. He talks like he's under strain. "Why doesn't he talk louder," I'd wonder. He stopped talking altogether. Neither one of us was smart enough to know anything about it. He still has that major problem today.

SHE: My voice is gone. I can still talk, but I've got to think about it to talk loud. I make a conscious effort.

When I'm walking, my gait is wonderful. It's the small steps in small areas and the turning that I have to talk myself through. Once I get going, I'm fine. When I'm "off," I get rigid and stiff and my feet get stuck, like freezing. I kind of kick my feet and say, "left, right, left, right," a trick to make myself move better. Once I start moving and walking around it goes away.

I have leg cramps, but I used to have them a whole lot worse. I used to be up all night, but they've subsided. The biggest problem right now is getting up out of a chair. I can't sit for too long. It's hard to turn to get up. I do an exercise where you cross your arms across your chest and push onto your heels.

I do some exercise every day, and I do the treadmill three times a week. I do them right here in the living room, or downstairs where we have a workout room.

HE: She exercises a lot.

SHE: The more I do, the better I can move. I've got to keep doing it. Fatigue is a terrible thing. A lot of times in the morning, by the time I get everything done, I'm really tired. Just getting ready – taking a shower, washing my hair, fixing breakfast, and doing the dishes.

HE: I think she has internal tremors, too. I look at her when she tells me she has dyskinesia. I can't see it, but she can feel it internally.

SHE: I have dyskinesia. You can tell I have it because I'm just moving all the time. It's the medication. I was with my daughter-in-law the other day and I got dyskinesia. I felt bad for her. We were in a restaurant and another table was watching us because I was shaking so badly. We were under very stressful conditions. She got me a regular Pepsi, even though I never drink caffeinated pop. The first swallow and the dyskinesia stopped. It was amazing. I figured it was the caffeine that worked.

I find that sometimes I drool when I'm sleeping. I have a problem with choking, but I concentrate and am very careful and conscious of what I eat.

My husband has been doing the paperwork for years. If I really concentrate, I think I could probably write.

HE: She has small writing. She'll start out and it will trail off to nothing.

SHE: I've noticed since my last appointment with the eye doctor last year, I can't read some of the stuff on the T.V.

HE: I think she has all kinds of eye problems. I've read that with Parkinson's, a lot of problems show up in your eyes. She's had cataracts removed, and more often than not, you're able to see better, but not in her case. Then she went to a retina specialist and had all of that stuff done. She still wears glasses, and even the glasses don't help her that much. The ophthalmologist doesn't see anything wrong.

SHE: Another thing happened. I just got attacked by a dog the day before Thanksgiving. He tore me all apart. He threw me to the ground, and he cracked my pelvis. I had to go to a hand specialist. They thought I'd lose the use of my right hand. I didn't.

HE: We're at the point where, sometimes, it's very difficult for her to get out and move. She doesn't like talking about this. She likes to think she can do everything and anything. The truth is, she just can't move. The walker doesn't help at those times. I think her meds work only 65-70% of the time. She's on a regimen where she takes her first meds whenever she gets up in the morning, and then every three hours after that. Even though she takes her meds on time, she goes "off" in 2 ½ hours, and sometimes she takes her meds and they don't kick in at all. She can't move. She can't walk.

SHE: Sometimes I can miss taking it by two hours and I don't even notice. But, sometimes if I go "off," it's hard to get back "on." We've been going to the specialist for quite a while. I take notes, and I listen to some of the stuff he tells me, and then another time he'll switch gears and tell me something different. I come home from my doctor's appointment upset. I've been upset for six years.

HE: The reason we go back is, how many specialists are there to go to? She has been upset every time she goes to the doctor. He looks at her in a condescending way. Now I kind of talk a little bit for her.

SHE: One time I talked to my doctor about my meds. "About 11:30 p.m. I'm 'off,'" I said. His response was, "Are you expecting to close the bars?"

I worry about the future a lot. I worry that I won't be able to live alone. My husband was just in the hospital. My daughter-in-law came to stay with me. I'm concerned because we've got this big house now. I just think, "What should we do? Sell the house and get something different? But, I enjoy the house. I never thought I'd be at this stage of Parkinson's. I knew it was degenerative, but I always thought I'd be OK. I wonder what it would be like if I was in a wheelchair.

HE: I know there's no set path.   Each patient is different.   I asked the doctor what percentage of patients end up in a wheelchair. He said, "Very few."

SHE: I was an x-ray technician, but mostly I was raising five kids. We've been married 52 years. We have 11 grandkids.

HE: I'm an engineer and a retired vice president of manufacturing operations for an automotive company. I worked there 30 years.

SHE: The children are conscious I have Parkinson's disease, but for a long time we just got on with our lives and didn't talk about it.

HE: That was kind of bad stuff when she first started with this Parkinson's thing. I didn't give it more than 20 seconds thought during the whole day. She said, "You'd better get smart about this Parkinson's." Once I realized what it was all about, I can't believe I had my head in the sand so much. In the early days, I could have given her more support. It was a major mistake on my behalf. And, she never complains about anything.

SHE: I still continue doing most everything I've always done.   But, I have to really work at it. My biggest problem to cope with is managing my day's activities around my medications so I won't be freezing up or too stiff. I have to try to be "on." If I am "off," I can't move very well. "On" is when I'm functioning pretty normally. "Off" is when I can't manage too well. I don't want to be "off" when I go to church or have an appointment.   What's getting bad for me is my meds aren't lasting that long, and when they don't, I can't move.

I don't get anything done unless I concentrate on doing one thing at a time. I can't multitask. I try to stay in the bedroom until I'm finished doing what I'm doing. If I go into the kitchen, I get off track. I know I can't do things like I did before. It's like being on a teeter-totter.

I was born in the country, one of nine kids. My mother died when I was 13. I had to help run the household. We just did what we had to do. My husband and I met at the drive-in movie when I was 23. He was in a family of nine kids, too.

My interests are mostly the kids and the family. We've been boating for 20 or 30 years. Our boat sleeps eight. It's like another home. It's hard to give it up because the kids have grown up on it.

I don't golf anymore. I used to sew. I re-upholstered all the furniture in my house once.

When we attend the support group, I just feel part of them, no matter who it is. I'd like to have a talk session. I try for us to get there early. That's why I go – to talk to people. That's how I learn.

HE: Once you have Parkinson's symptoms, learn as much as you can about the disease so you'll know what to expect and are not surprised and depressed. Bring your caregiver into the loop immediately so they'll become cognizant of what you're going through. Make it a team effort.

SHE: I cope by trusting the Lord. I just thank the Lord I'm alive, and I concentrate on the beautiful world I live in – beautiful family, beautiful friends.

My advice would be to keep a smile on your face. Pray hard. If I'm laughing, I feel a lot, lot better. Try to associate with happy people. It's unbelievable how much better I feel when I'm just having a good time. You don't need to be serious all your life.

IT'S NOT A DISEASE – IT'S AN INCONVENIENCE

AGE: 76
DIAGNOSED: 17 years
HE: Parkinson's Patient
SHE: Spouse

HE: For about 15 years after I was diagnosed with Parkinson's disease (PD), I didn't really exhibit many symptoms. The last two years, however, many things have kind of burst into being. Now others would know I have Parkinson's disease by looking at me.

SHE: You couldn't tell he had Parkinson's until about two years ago. Now he leans to one side. Sometimes he walks a little slow.

HE: Back about 17 1/2 years ago, I was walking to work one day with a briefcase in my hand. I dropped it. I picked it up again, but I couldn't hold onto it. At that particular time, I thought I had a problem. I started going to a series of doctors, and sure enough, I did have a problem.

SHE: In the very beginning, the first six months, people would ask, "What's wrong. Does he have cancer?" They didn't know, and he didn't tell them. He was 58 years old.

HE: My voice changed. It was erratic and it wasn't loud enough for people to hear me. I look back and realize that I first noticed it at business meetings. It was hard to communicate with my fellow salesmen. The secretary where I worked suggested I might have Parkinson's, but I didn't look into it until I starting shuffling and freezing.

SHE: When I first met him and when we were dating, he had a stare about him. I'd say, "Blink, honey, blink." Even though we saw all those signs, we didn't think anything of it. He even had the masking back then. When he was diagnosed, he didn't tell them at work, but they surmised he had Parkinson's. Not too long afterwards, they told him they had to downsize and he was the first person to go. When he retired and told everybody that he had Parkinson's, it was like he was a new man because of the relief. The stress of work and the stress of keeping the secret was taking a toll on him.

Michael J. Fox came out with his diagnosis about the same time. There was a big hoopla about him because he was so young. I do have one cute comment. In the very beginning, my husband didn't want to tell people because he didn't want people to hold on to him and help him. When others kept talking about his Parkinson's disease, he said, "It's not a disease. It's not contagious. It's just an inconvenience."

HE: When I was first diagnosed, I went to a clinic that treated people with PD. Then I went to a neurologist at a university hospital. She asked all kinds of irrelevant questions and was horrible. From there, someone recommended a movement specialist.

SHE: The diagnosis bothered him, but at the same time, he also found out he had a big hearing loss in both ears. He was more devastated about having to wear hearing aids.

HE: I have tremors when I'm very cold or when I'm facing an audience. My good friend and I put on an affair for a club. I wanted to thank all the people who helped with the party. My clipboard was shaking like crazy. My friend just took it and held it for me while I finished.

SHE: These last couple of years he has a heck of a time putting his coat on. I've also noticed a little bit of drooling on the side of his mouth. For a while there, he started to stand up straight, but he leans way to the left and down. The back doctor says it's Parkinson's, not a curvature of the spine. The doctor seems to attach a variety of symptoms to PD.

HE: I'm the PD poster boy with the dancing feet. My legs and my feet move all the time and I have to think about it to stop them.

SHE: Right now, they're shaking up a storm. His toes are curling under.

HE: I do a lot of shuffling. Usually, I start and stop and start and stop. Sometimes, I can break the pattern. I make a point. I say to myself, "I'm going to walk a normal pace." I have to psych myself up to move, and I have to plan my route. Typically, in a restaurant, if the restrooms are buried behind the kitchen, I look at the route first and think it through, because I don't want to fall over people – which I've done.

SHE: Sometimes his balance isn't that great, and he can be a little wobbly. The other thing is he also freezes a lot. Sometimes I just touch him and say, "OK, take a step."

HE: The last time I was frozen, I couldn't get out of bed.

SHE: It was horrible. I still don't think his meds are right. He drops a lot on the floor, and we don't know if he's taken them all. I honestly think he hasn't taken his pills right for a long time. We've got to find a different method to keep his medicine in order. We'd really like to see if our doctor can change them.

I'm looking at his body and can tell the way he's walking and acting that he's missed taking his pill. It takes a while to get him geared up again after he's missed. I ask him, "Can't you tell by the way you're walking and feeling that you've missed a dose?" It's a problem.

Sometimes I giggle at some of the things he comes up with, laughing over his own situation. Our oldest granddaughter is going to be 13. When she was born, the first time he held her in his arms, she started to cry. "Maybe with my shaking, I can rock her to sleep," he said.

HE: Recently I noticed that when I write little notes, I start out OK, but then I get sloppy and words become compressed looking. Even my signature is getting a little wiry.

SHE: Sometimes I'll ask him a question, and he doesn't answer me real quick. He needs a minute before he understands what I've said to him.

HE: It takes time for the question to sink in, for me to analyze it and to answer it.

SHE: Sometimes he can be very quiet. We'll tease him and say, "Don't talk so much."

HE: It's because I'm self-conscious and afraid I won't be heard anyway so I just shut my mouth. It makes me feel left out a little bit. I went to the BIG and LOUD speech therapy – a very good program. There are all kinds of things I can do, but I don't do them anymore. I don't exercise either on a regular basis. I should get out and walk. She does.

I use a walker in the night to walk to the bathroom. I keep a walking stick in the car, and I have a handicap sticker on the mirror. I use them if the weather is bad, or if it's a long distance to where we're going, or if I have to walk on the grass. I make that judgment call when I see the situation. I get paranoid around stairs. If we go to someone's house where there are a lot of them, she helps me and I use the stick. We went to a hockey game and our seats were on the third tier. It was frightening coming down. I depended on someone to grab onto my left elbow while I used the stick in the other hand; or I'll use the railing first.

I like to keep up my skills of driving, but I do drive slower, and I can't drive at night. She's a better driver and does a lot of the driving.

Getting in and out of bed is terrible. Mostly it's getting in.

SHE: It takes us a while to get him into bed. He gets in and has his head and his shoulder on the bed. I wouldn't mind getting him satin sheets so he could slide into bed, but then he'd slide right out. He's pretty rigid. He doesn't relax, even when he lies down.

He's had problems with constipation, but that's taken care of.

He has dreams, but the only time he had hallucinations was when he was in the hospital with his back operation. He was on their "pain cocktail," morphine. He hallucinated for three days.

When he's in the closet too long, it dawns on me that he's probably trying to button his shirt. He's very patient. I have to try to buy shirts without buttons.

He had perfect teeth, but with all the medications, his teeth are not as healthy as they used to be.

HE: I don't eat large quantities of food, and I eat goodies between meals.

SHE: He does lose weight because of not eating. He wants dinner, but he only eats a little bit. He has a problem cutting his meat and eating spaghetti and soup. Every time he eats his spaghetti, I think of the cartoon, *Lady and the Tramp.*

We've had a lot of nice trips since we've been married and he's always had Parkinson's, but it's getting harder, especially if it involves walking. A couple of small cruises worked out well.

HE: I feel I have to get over this shuffling bit, and it's going to take some work.

SHE: He gets so focused on whatever it is he's doing. Once he has a project, he can't focus on having lunch, or sitting and resting, or anything else.

When we first dated, he would think of a lot of fun and different things to do. "I'm just not an ordinary penguin," he told me. He always had creative ideas, and when he did something, he went beyond to do something unusual. Now I have to come up with the ideas.

HE: I like to be different and go upstream, not downstream.

SHE: Everything he does is with a different twist. When we were sailing, he ordered a new boat and he wanted the deck to be painted caramel. The boat maker sent him colors to choose from. He finally said, "This is not the right color caramel." So, he crushed a caramel candy and stuck it in an envelope and mailed it to them and said, "This is caramel." He got what he wanted, and combined with black, the boat was a standout as it sailed around the club.

HE: We used to be quite the dancers. This year, we just slow danced at the gala. I was concerned about stumbling. We are involved as co-chairmen for entertainment, or whatever else is needed for the annual Parkinson's gala. We're involved in our support group, too, and I think the best thing it does is bring new thoughts and ideas to the general meeting. It's a way of keeping us up to date with what's happening, and what drugs are available for Parkinson's.

SHE: I'm amazed how much I learn from our leader and from the caregiver's group. A lot of ladies are in the same boat as me, and we help one another accept what is, since we can't change it. When I go to support groups, I don't find that people with Parkinson's are bitter, nor do I see very many people break apart their marriage.

We know the Parkinson's is always going to be there. Like anyone, he can get some real down days, but he's learned to let go of a lot of things. He was such a tense person. I tell him, "The most important thing you have to do today is take care of you." It puts everything into perspective.

HE: I look beyond that day and see what's coming up in the future, something I'm looking forward to. Parkinson's is progressive. There's no cure for it. You have to accept what it is and get on with your life. We get a handicapped sticker. When we fly, we go to the front of the line, with a wheelchair. And we get to be the first ones to board. That's a good thing.

KEEP DOING WHAT YOU DID FOR AS LONG AS YOU CAN

AGE: 68
DIAGNOSED: 18 years
Male Parkinson's Patient

Now, everyday stuff is aggravating. I have motor skill problems, psychological problems, and social problems. My body will keep going, but my feet won't. Back then, the first aggravating problems I noticed were that I couldn't put my jacket on, and I had to switch arms to fish.

I went to our primary doctor who diagnosed me with Parkinson's disease (PD) immediately and sent me to a neurologist. I was diagnosed by a neurologist at age 50.

I was sad and resentful because I had taken care of myself. I exercised, ate good food, and didn't drink or smoke. I was very athletic and always snow skied with the kids, had boats, and played golf. It was hard to give up my boat, but it became too confining. We now have a 24 foot pontoon boat, and that's perfect.

I was getting dyskinesia about five years ago. I did the DBS surgery in 2008. It was recommended by my doctor, a movement specialist, who believes in quality of life.

The surgery helped the dyskinesia a lot. I don't shake anymore. My doctor's philosophy is to stay on as low a dosage of meds as possible.

For a long time I didn't notice, but I believe protein blocks the effectiveness of the meds.

I have hallucinations, not real bad, like borderline screaming out in the night.

I feel like we've been around the block for 18 years with this thing. But, it's so individual. It's been said, it is so many diseases in one. If I didn't have a good caregiver, I'd be stuck in a chair somewhere.

The biggest frustration is my inability to just get into the car and drive to a fishing spot. I still drive, but not far. I'm afraid of getting stuck. The less mobility I have, the more alone I feel.

One of my favorite things to do is to go salmon fishing in the fall. Two of the guys I've been going with for 40 years pick me up and take me with them. It's a very pretty spot, very calming and meditative. Otherwise, we're not always included anymore with friends for weekend outings or other travels. I think we cramp their style because of my schedule.

The Parkinson's support group has been a great group for knowledge and for sharing with one another. What is so great about being in the support group is you see other people dealing with PD, too.

I was exposed to chemicals from my grandpa's apple orchard where I often went from ages five to fifteen. I also served in Vietnam at age 21.

I worked at least 30 years in Information Technology and was very good on the computer. I still use the computer a lot. I worked on the big ones, though.

This disease "whacks" me real fast, but I don't take a nap or rest much. I'm better off if I keep moving, because once I stop, I can't start.

Our one-arm golfing buddy beats us at golf. I want some of his meds.

[See his spouse's story on the following pages.]

HE IS AN INSPIRATION

Female Spouse

You can tell my husband has a lack of facial expression, and he doesn't talk loud enough for people to hear him. Talking takes a lot of energy.

He used to walk a lot. When we went for walks together, I asked him why his arm wasn't swinging. On his 50th birthday, he walked five miles around the lake, a goal he had set. After he finished his walk, he didn't feel very well. After five years of noticing unusual symptoms and wondering what was wrong, I said, "Maybe you should have these things checked out." That's when he finally went to the doctor.

Of course, we were in shock when he was diagnosed with Parkinson's disease (PD). We knew nothing about PD or the long-term effects of it. If we'd known, we may have cried, but we didn't know. After the shock wore off, we thought, "This isn't so bad," even though the prognosis looked terrible from the research we did.

My husband said, "I might as well eat hamburgers." Prior to that, he took better care of his health than all his friends, who were overweight. I think he's been able to do more, though, because of his good, healthy habits.

I remember the doctor saying he'd have ten good years, and he has. He's lived a long time "normally." After ten years, the doctor said he'd have another good ten years, but over time, he's gotten worse, and the disease is slowly taking things away from us. I try to keep us busy. He'll get up and empty the wastebasket just to have something to do.

I think the biggest thing with Parkinson's is getting the meds regulated. There have been a lot of changes the last month with generic meds coming in. He was doing fine on non-generic, but since we switched to all generic, he's having problems. He gets burning, stiff muscles in his legs. We think it is the meds, anyway.

We're going to have to go back to the doctor and get non-generic.

The hardest thing for me is that our social life is suffering. He feels lonesome if I go out and do things, but I do bridge, water aerobics, water colors, and acrylics. We live on a lake and he fishes a lot.

By 7:30 p.m., he's done for the night. We never know how he'll feel at the end of the day. That's the worst time for him. For the last eight years, his meds might shut off anytime, and he gets rigid and unable to move.

Our two children live out of state. We really have enjoyed doing things with the grandchildren, but at Christmas, he said he was feeling sad that he couldn't play with them much because he couldn't move very well. And, with all the noise and confusion, he freezes up.

I think people may see someone with Parkinson's and think, "They seem OK," but they have no clue what the PD person is struggling with, and how hard it is for them to manage. I think there are personality changes, too. It's hard for my husband to feel happy. He gets depressed and I think he ends up feeling alone and lonely because people can't hear him when he talks. Nevertheless, many people, especially all the guys at the golf course, say to me, "He's an inspiration because he keeps going."

We love the support of the PD support group, but we can't go at night anymore. After about 7:30 p.m., he's done for the evening. We go to the monthly breakfasts and other events.

He can't sit too long. He's constantly shifting in his chair. He burned up a lot of calories and lost a lot of weight because his body was constantly moving. He freezes up and can't move if I'm waiting for him. He tells me to leave the room. Or, he freezes up if his golfing buddies are waiting for him. It must make him stressed.

He's on meds that can prompt compulsive behavior. He does like to go to the casinos, but his behavior is not out of control. The doctors try to stay away from increasing his meds for as long as possible. I don't think the doctor tells us enough, though. "Take this. See you in six months," and you go home feeling depressed. We have suffered a lot, trying to work through all the issues with certain meds that bothered him. He'd fall on the floor and I couldn't move him. He gets off balance easily, or his feet stick and he falls forward. He's been stiffening up with pain. It's a constant battle. I've learned to schedule an appointment two weeks out when his meds are changed, or his DBS reprogrammed. That way, we can evaluate the affects, instead of waiting another six months.

He has all the latest technology, having been in the business – an iPad, iPhone, PC, and laptop. In our 37 years of marriage, we've never had a repairman in our house. My husband can do it all. We had a water main break in our house a couple of weeks ago. The basement was flooded almost immediately. Though he can hardly move by himself, he had it fixed by the end of the day. You could call him "a friendly helper;" a do-it-yourself, independent guy. He never was and still isn't a guy that leans on his wife to do everything. He's a good friend and an excellent father. He likes to travel to see our family. He'd like to do more as a grandfather. We've explained to our grandchildren the effects of the meds on him. It's given them compassion. They'll say sometimes, "Grandpa's legs don't work very well now. Does he need his meds?"

We keep him on a good schedule, but lately he's been grouchy. His leg hurts. He had two stents put in when he was having DBS surgery in 2008. That's when they discovered 100% blockage in one artery – another hurdle to deal with.

We've been together for 44 years. We were high school sweethearts. Our family has been active in sports. He was a soccer coach for seven years and always had a winning team. We always loved to travel and took our children many places in the U.S. and Canada.

I taught second grade for many years and retired six years ago.

A friend of ours was diagnosed with PD last year. He quit playing golf because he was embarrassed to play in front of his friends. My husband didn't quit. His friends drive the cart right up to the ball for him, and they pick it up for him when needed. It gives other people a chance to help him and makes him realize you can live with something if you put your mind to it. He pushes negative thoughts out of his mind. I'd be a lot more depressed if I were him. He keeps positive thoughts in his head, and lives one day at a time. Many people have told me he is an inspiration to them. He never complains, and he keeps going. He says, "This is how Parkinson's is. I am not going to be embarrassed about it. You can still live your life and think about what you can do, rather than what you can't do."

I do the driving when we go to Florida where the sunshine makes him feel better, and he doesn't have to worry about slipping on the ice. He tells me, jokingly, "I know I'm old now, because I got a metal detector for scanning the beaches for diamond rings and doubloons." He's an optimistic guy. Let's hope he finds more than bottle caps.

FRIENDSHIPS HAVE HELPED ME THE MOST

AGE: 65
DIAGNOSED: 44 years
Female Parkinson's Patient

During my last year of college, I started to shake. I shook all over. My gait slowed down. I couldn't keep up with other students walking across campus. The worst thing of all was having people tell me to stop shaking when I couldn't. And, people trying to diagnose me with multiple sclerosis, or something else.

I went to a local neurologist, but ended up at a university clinic with a diagnosis of Parkinson's disease (PD). To get Parkinson's at that age was really unusual. I was only 21. The news was devastating. My grandmother had Parkinson's. By observing her, I knew it was something I didn't want.

I had gone to college for four years and I wanted to get a job, in spite of my diagnosis. I wasn't going to give up. I interviewed for a teaching position. My doctor said to me one day, "Do you know how bright you are?" That comment gave me enough confidence to go on. He talked to the administrators of the school system. He asked if they were aware of my condition. Whatever he said to them, they must have accepted, because they never questioned my ability. I was hired as a teacher for the first, second, and third grades in a small school. I will always be grateful to the school administration for accommodating my health problems. It was never hard to do my lessons, and I wasn't handicapped interacting with the kids. If I had to leave the room because of a tremor, the other teachers would take over for me. My tremors were full body tremors. I would shake all over. To stop them, I'd go to a place until I could calm them down and get relaxed.

There are other symptoms. On one visit to a doctor, I overheard him tell someone in his office that my face was "expressionless." My handwriting was small and scribbly. I also continued to be stiff. I found it hard to walk up inclines. Sometimes my whole body would shake from the tremors, so much so that I'd go to the emergency room. They didn't know what to do with me because they didn't know that much about Parkinson's.

To keep informed, I received information from the Parkinson foundation. I read about a new medicine. I told my doctor I wanted to take it. "You can take it, but don't expect miracles," he said. The medicine came with no instructions. I had to figure out how to take it by reading information the Parkinson foundation sent me. Back then, the medicine came only in dosages of 10/100. When I took it, it was like a miracle to me. I could walk up the incline, which only a month earlier I had difficulty with.

By 1992, I was becoming quite fatigued and my dyskinesia was bad. I was alarmed by the fact that the dyskinesia was caused by too much of one of my medications. No one would wish those movements to be a part of their life. My doctor gave me a letter saying he felt that I couldn't keep up with the physical duties of my job.

For about ten years after I retired, I stayed home because of my tremors. I had them every two hours and they were severe. I developed depression – a part of the disease. I didn't leave the house because of panic disorder. With the help of my psychiatrist, I was able to overcome the panic and get on with my life.

When you've had Parkinson's for 40 years, you've been through it all. I started on drugs in the 1970s. I tried all the newest drugs as they came on the market. I've been in the hospital several times, had different doctors, and done drug trials.

On my way to church one day I hit a curb when turning and got a flat tire. That's when I decided I didn't want to drive anymore. I didn't want to hurt other people. I kept my car and hired someone to drive me around from time to time. I was retired by then. I've also had an agency come to my home and help me with errands. I still have a girl today that I've had over the years. I do feel trapped, not driving, but for safety reasons, I don't want to. The Secretary of State won't give me a license because of my dyskinesia. I jerk the car when I'm driving.

Walking is my biggest handicap because I walk on my toes. I try to work out walking strategies. I'm always thinking, heel first. Otherwise, my walk is like a hop. To this day, I still hesitate with my right foot when I try to walk. I think, "Am I walking normally? Am I picking up my feet enough? Am I shuffling? Am I having dyskinesia? Am I freezing?" These thoughts continually cross my mind. I spend so much time thinking about how I'll walk across a room, out to the mailbox, or into the next room. This continual analysis takes all the joy out of life. It makes things a lot easier if I just accept that this is just who I am.

Ten years ago, because my dyskinesia was really bad, I interviewed with a Deep Brain Stimulation (DBS) specialist. It wasn't until six years ago that I went ahead with the surgery. It's worked. I'm glad I had it. I feel like this is the best adjusted I've been in my life, physically and emotionally. I don't have ups and downs like I used to have before DBS. I'm not saying it's a cure, because I still have trouble walking, but I'm more confident than I used to be. I have less anxiety. I haven't been shaking. My tremors are hardly noticeable. Now, I can do more things like painting and sewing and be involved with a service club I belong to. I also helped found our local Parkinson's disease support group.

In the past, I had experienced "On" and "Off" times with my medication. After DBS, I was committed to taking as little medicine as possible. I started taking half tablets and quarter tablets closer together, instead of a whole tablet further apart. I wanted to keep a balanced amount in my system.

Once, after the DBS surgery, I had a bad experience. On a doctor's visit, I had turned off my stimulators to have an EKG. I thought I had turned them back on. The tremors came back on one side. I couldn't straighten myself out. I called the head of our local support group and she came over to check my stimulators. She found that I had only turned one side back on. What an experience. It was very upsetting. It took me another day to calm down.

I went to the first Parkinson's disease congress in D.C. ten years ago. That was my first time to travel. The same year, I went to Atlanta for a national Parkinson's disease conference. I've visited my brother in Florida. To travel, it takes me time to prepare right. I also use the wheelchair at the airport.

I would advise others with symptoms to get a doctor that's a movement disorder specialist. Together, figure out the proper dosage of your medicines. There was a period of time they didn't know much about the drugs and I was on my own to experiment. They've learned a lot about Parkinson's and the drugs in the last 20 years.

My advice would be, don't give up. Keep yourself busy. Find a Parkinson's support group. We share our experiences in our support group and we find solutions for things. One girl shared that she used toe separators for her toe spasms, so I got them for myself. Because my toes are close together, it's painful. The toe separators help. It's the small things that mean a lot.

Parkinson's disease has guided my whole life since I was 20. The hardest thing to cope with has been the tremors. They wore me out, they were so bad. Since DBS surgery, I don't have them. From time to time, I have fears of falling. I still take an anti-depressant.

I've been exercising twice a day for two years now, and I'm convinced that without it, I wouldn't be walking around. I do a combination of "BIG" exercises, the stationary bike, shoulder shrugs, and yoga balance exercises.

I live alone. I have to count on myself to be motivated, and to plan my future. I think it's a good thing, because I've developed coping skills and have become a problem-solver.

Friendships, along with having the right doctors and the right meds, have helped me the most. I knew my friend/caregiver for a long time before I realized he had a Ph.D. from the University of Michigan. He also served in the medical corps in Europe.

[See her friend/caregiver's story on the following pages.]

I'M INSPIRED BY HER COURAGE AND DETERMINATION

Male Friend/Caregiver

I've been in the Parkinson's support group since the beginning. I was one of the original four founders.

I met her 20 years ago. I was in private practice at the time, and she was referred to me by her neurologist. At the time, I was a clinical psychologist. She became a client of mine. My assessment was that hers was a work-related "adjustment disorder." It was not Parkinson's related. She was probably 40 years old at the time and still teaching.

She had been diagnosed with Parkinson's disease (PD) shortly after her senior year in college. I didn't know much about Parkinson's. I thought, "My gosh, how nervous this person is." She had tremors. My clinical training did not include therapy for individuals with chronic health problems. However, I could help her with the use of relaxation techniques and could provide her with some degree of support.

One day she called me up and said she had to see her neurologist at Henry Ford Hospital, but she didn't have any way to get there. I drove her to the hospital and drove into the parking garage. She started to tremor. The tremors were intense. I hadn't noticed it in therapy. It reminded me of a seizure. I felt so helpless. She said, "There's nothing you can do. We'll just wait it out." That's what we did.

I had noticed during the therapy sessions that her social life was very isolated. Her life consisted of working, going home to grade papers, and cleaning her house on weekends.

She does not have strong family support, so I decided to go outside the therapy sessions to break down her social isolation. I took her to art museums and art exhibits. I encouraged her to take up her art again. She's quite an artist. I suggested that she return to church. She could drive when I first met her, but that ended. Now, she has caregivers assisting her.

Once we went outside the office, it was unorthodox in terms of treatment. It was voluntary on my part. I've been doing it all these years as a friend.

Her tremors became increasingly worse and interfered with her work. She had dyskinesia more often and more intense, so she retired with a disability.

I continue to take her to her doctors' appointments because they appreciate my observations. All this gets interrupted when I go south every winter for three months. But I've called her every Saturday to see how she is doing. She's really an inspiring person. I enjoy her company. At times, I thought, "What the hell am I doing?" because I felt so helpless.

I'm married and have six kids. She never married nor had children. The only family she has is a brother in Florida.

Because of my relationship with her, I called the Michigan Parkinson Foundation about seven years ago, inquiring about support groups. There were none out this way. I know how valuable they are. I went to the local hospital and made arrangements to set one up. The Michigan Parkinson Foundation took it from there by notifying neurologists that we were starting a new support group. I think the foundation got someone else involved with her as co-facilitators.

I also got her involved in a service club which focuses on people with developmental disabilities. She takes notes for that club. She is secretary at a church women's group. All that is possible because she had the DBS surgery. She's come a long way.

The DBS surgery changed things remarkably. It was like a miracle. The tremors stopped and the dyskinesia stopped. When I was first involved with her, not much was known about DBS surgery. They only had one drug for PD. They didn't focus on anything but the tremors. Now we also have the BIG and LOUD programs (LSVT) for strengthening the voice and encouraging bigger movements.

I attend all the Parkinson's support groups except when I'm in Florida. I've given a couple of talks to the *Living with Parkinson's Disease* group and other groups. I've certainly gained a lot of knowledge in the last 20 years, but my feeling is that there's so much I don't know. The brain is so complex and interrelated. The symptoms are diverse, and there are many varieties of the disease. That's what makes finding a cure so difficult.

At first, anyone would have known there was something wrong by her tremors. And, her voice is very quiet. I often have to ask her to speak louder. Now, it's pretty obvious by the way she walks. Her walking has become increasingly impaired. It's not exactly flat-footed. Her toes come down first instead of her heel. She takes real short steps. Sometimes she shuffles. Before the walker, she shuffled a lot. She has used a walker for the last two years.

She has other characteristics of a person with Parkinson's, like when she becomes immobile and freezes. Occasionally, the body stiffens when the body is in motion. She developed dyskinesia from too much medication. The dyskinesia is the out of control, random movements of the body. She stoops occasionally.

It's very important that a caregiver learn as much as they can about the disease and be cautious about what they do for the person. I would encourage the one with Parkinson's to speak up and tell the caregiver what to do and what not to do. Otherwise, they're being helped with things they should be doing for themselves.

Of prime importance for the caregiver is to have a life separate from the Parkinson's patient. Have your own hobbies. Otherwise, you'll end up with resentment, guilt, and stress related illnesses. It's normal for a caregiver to feel put upon sometime. If you don't take care of yourself, you can't take care of anyone. Our support group does quite a bit for caregivers.

I have a wide variety of interests. I have a wonderful wife, have great grandchildren, and attend their events. I love fishing, and I love to read. I volunteer at a mental health clinic. At 84, I can still drive. I can still carry on a conversation like this. I'm not a full-time caregiver. I see her three hours a week, at most.

I believe our purpose in life is to serve others, so I do whatever I can. Spending time with someone is one way to serve. My wife is very accepting of my involvement with many different things. I do the Parkinson's walkathon. I have a service club which helps the developmentally disabled.

Being involved has increased my sense of gratefulness. Seeing people struggle with Parkinson's disease gives me an appreciation and a compassion for others. I'd like to say, as a caregiver, I can't help but be inspired by the courage and determination of people with Parkinson's. I think it is important for them to remember that there's so much hope for the future, so much progress being made.

God brings certain people into our life. If I hadn't met her, I wouldn't be involved with Parkinson's.

HE SET A GOOD EXAMPLE

AGE: 75 AT DEATH
Widowed Spouse

He was 75 when he died. He was officially diagnosed with Parkinson's disease (PD) in his early 60s, but he had it for about five years before that.

He was such a healthy, active man. From the time I met him he always ate right, exercised, and did all the right things. He only had an occasional social drink and he did not smoke. He was a jogger, a cyclist, and had a boat. He had a physically demanding job. As branch manager and overseer for a construction company, he had to climb scaffolding and he travelled extensively.

He was always happy. He really never felt sorry for himself. From the time he was diagnosed, he set a good example to carry on with life and make the best of it.

He said to me one day, "I can't smell anything. I don't know what's going on with me." I said, "Oh, that's silly." He would often mention, "You know, I can't remember things like I used to." He had always been sharp, remembering every detail. Then he said, "I think I better retire." He took an early retirement. One day he said, "I can't get my legs and feet to move like they should."

I've been in the nursing field for 30 years. I worked full time for a group of orthopedic surgeons, so I said to them, "My husband is complaining he can't move his legs and feet like he used to." They said, "Bring him in and let us look at him." They had him walk down the hall. By then I noticed that he was walking differently, holding his hands to his side. They both looked at each other and they looked at me and said, "We suspect he has Parkinson's disease based on the background you've given us and our observations." They said, "You need to go to a neurologist." The neurologist tested his reflexes, his walk, and his strength. He said the same thing, "I really feel you have PD," so he started him on medication. After three years, and seeing him every three months, he said, "You know, I'm really not a Parkinson's doctor. I would feel more comfortable if you would go to a specialist in that field."

Even though my husband is gone from me now, there are times I still hear his shuffling. I would be in another part of the house, and if he wanted me, he would get up and shuffle his feet.

My husband had some masking, his posture had changed, he had that rigid stance about him, and he was stooped. He also had problems remembering. The doctor would say, "I'm going to give you four words now, and I want you to remember these because I'm going to come back to them." And later, "Alright, do you remember those four words?" The more advanced he got into Parkinson's, the less he could remember those four words. It was impossible for him to tap his fingertips together and tap his feet.

He had to give up jogging long before this. He was an avid biker. For years he would go on those "Peddle across Michigan" bike tours where they would bike for about five days. After his PD, he could get on the bike and ride it, but if he had to stop on the trail, he would fall. I would come home from work many times and he'd be sitting there all bloody because he had fallen off the bike. I'd have to take him to the hospital for stitches for a cut lip or a cut forehead.

He was more in tune with Parkinson's than I was. When I came into the family in the early 60s, his father was really battling PD and I, of course, observed this, but I never in my wildest dreams thought it would affect us. At the time, his father was stooped, had a rigid walk, and was drooling. He had a bad tremor, and the last two years of his life, he was a vegetable. He had to be taken care of totally by my mother-in-law. He was dependent on her for everything. My husband and I talked about this and he said, "I hope I never get like my father was." I said, "I don't think you will, because there are meds on the market now that weren't then."

I feel his medication did help him greatly, but he already had dementia by the time he went to the neurologist. He said, "I just can't remember things like I should."

I retired because I knew I had to be home with him. I knew I couldn't trust him alone.

When he died, the only thing he could do physically was take our seven pound poodle for a short walk. It was on a Saturday evening. I had picked up our three-year-old granddaughter to come here for pizza and to make chocolate chip cookies. He was sitting in his chair laughing at us. He said, "I think I had better take the dog for a walk." The next thing I know, there was a neighbor at my door saying, "I think you'd better come." He had fallen and had a head injury and nothing could be done to stop the bleeding. The next day he went into a coma and he died six days later.

He had Sundowners so bad. At sunset, he would switch off just like a light switch. He couldn't control anything. I'd have to physically lay on him so he would stay in bed. I was monitoring his meds to see if there was something working against him. We called the ambulance many times. They had a tough time dealing with him. He said, "I've got to go fight the civil war in Virginia."

The PD specialist is very knowledgeable about PD, but his personality – he wouldn't really talk to us. He wouldn't tell us what the heck PD was all about. "Oh, he's still about stage three," he would say. I knew darn well his condition had gotten worse.

When the doctor didn't want him driving any more, he was ready to change doctors, but I wanted him off the road because he was falling asleep when driving. He was tested at the Secretary of State, and they took his driver's license away. That didn't make him very happy, but it did me.

He had trouble getting up. He was very stiff. I bought him a lift chair several years ago so he could sit up and get out of his chair. It would push him up so he would be almost standing.

You could barely hear him when he spoke. It would be like if you were talking to a three year old who was shy and not outgoing. He refused to use a walker. He shuffled. The doctor said, "You are such a physical person in such good physical condition, I think it's going to help you in your fight." But, unfortunately, what helped take him down was a heart attack a year before he died. He had to have stents put in, and then he had a couple of strokes. It didn't completely immobilize him, but his speech was affected. He stuttered and it took him a couple of minutes to get his thoughts out.

He loved to read books on World War II, but it became impossible for him to read with his bad eyesight. The eye doctor tested him and told him his eyes were OK, but he kept saying, "I just can't see." I never thought too much about that, but he had cataract surgery two years ago.

It was hard getting in and out of a car, into and out of bed without help, and getting around day to day. I would take him to the store with me because, in the end, I couldn't leave him alone. I'd sit him down and say, "Just sit here. I'll come and get you when I'm done." That helped get him out more and we would have a meal together while we were out.

He had constipation from all the medications. That's pretty common with Parkinson's meds. He constantly dabbed at his drippy nose. I took over and did most of the writing. He couldn't walk without veering. I had to put his socks on and his shoes. Swallowing and chewing was becoming more difficult. He choked. It scared me, especially when he was lying down.

He had hallucinations for about four years before his meds were changed. He'd say, "There's someone here in the house. We've got to find out what's going on." He didn't sleep well. When he did sleep, it was not a sound sleep. He started hallucinating and he would physically hurt me, kicking me, or leaning over my face, ready to start pounding me. He had no idea. I got myself away from him. I called the PD doctor the next day and I took him in. He put him on an anti-psychotic medication that controlled the hallucinations.

I saw his degeneration. I kept telling my kids – one daughter is a doctor – "I can see the changes are coming fast and I'm getting a little concerned here." She agreed with me. "Mom, I think you ought to go to another doctor," which I did.

My husband would complain, "You know, there's just something going on. I can't explain it. I don't know what's happening to me." I think it was the effect of PD on his whole body. He complained about his shoulders, but his legs and feet were more of a problem than his shoulders. He had always taken care of his teeth, but there was a problem. They were going bad. He had difficulty brushing them, so I bought him an electric tooth brush where all he had to do was push a button. He couldn't blink. He would kind of stare at me. In the last days of his life, he probably wasn't seeing much. When he finally finished that last book and laid it down, I think he was at his end.

He had the claw-effect of both his hands. He would grab a utensil to eat like a child does. Chewing was difficult, and I had to shred his meat into small pieces.

Knowing what his mother went through, I had depression and anger from the get-go. It was hard seeing him go from the healthy, positive man that he was, to a man suffering like his father did. I said, "What am I headed for?" But, I was with him 49 years and I certainly loved him and knew it was my job to be with him to the end. We often discussed that very thing. He would say, "I'm no good to you or anyone else." I told him, "You've always been the best thing that came into my life and you're loved and I will be with you and take care of you."

To cope, I found it very comforting to go into my back bedroom and meditate. The joy of our life has been our little granddaughter. I have been her caretaker since the get-go because my daughter teaches. She has her play room and papa would sit in his chair and talk and play with her.

We loved to walk in the park downtown. We would take our granddaughter to play. We belonged to the senior center, and we used to walk around the track and have lunch over there periodically.

About three years before he passed away, I started going to church. There were times I felt vulnerable, but I still had the comfort of knowing he was there. Now, I'm learning just how frightening it is to be alone, but I'm not going to give up. I'm happy that I have the connection with church and that I can go meditate and think about my life and what I'm going to do. It is difficult. I cope by just keeping myself busy. I have a sewing room downstairs. I like to make quilts. I couldn't do much before because I was caring for him.

Caring for the Parkinson's patient, I would suggest you learn as much as you can to be a good caregiver, but do not forget yourself. He was getting depressed at the end, and I was trying to be upbeat for him. As a caregiver for years, you are always talking about what you should be doing for the Parkinson's patient, never asking, "What about my needs?" never asking, "What would happen if I go first?" That was my biggest fear – what if I got sick and couldn't take care of him?

I met him in a little coffee shop. We both worked in the same building, he for the Corps of Engineers for the State, and me for the Better Business Bureau. We dated less than three months and we got married. We were married in 1963. He built houses on the side. He built our first house in 1968. We have four children.

I think people don't know how to respond to someone with Parkinson's. Friends didn't come around as much, and we didn't go out as much. He talked very slow and soft and tended to not say much. For that reason, he didn't want to go out anymore.

We went to the very first meeting of the newly-formed local Parkinson's support group in 2006. We met many good people. I've always enjoyed the PD support group throughout the years, having a place we can talk and share what is going on in our life, and helping others. Because of that support group, we learn a lot. We have a lot of guest speakers. This group really delves into problems and solutions. I think the Caregiver's group has really been important, too. One of the current facilitators and I went to one a long distance away. She said, "Let's see what we can do about starting our own," and we did.

Our four children are worried they might have the PD gene. It really concerns my son the most, because it seems like PD is more prevalent in men than women.

Something positive that has come out of this is that it makes us closer; it makes us appreciate each day that we have together. It makes the caregiver appreciate someone else who may be going through the same thing. I would say to the Parkinson's patient, try to stay as independent as you can. I would say to caregivers, just never give up and just cherish each day. Try to overlook a lot. Let the fire department and police station know about your situation in case you have to call on them. Let people know. Let your neighbors know. They'll watch out for you. They did for me.

...BUT I BROUGHT YOU FLOWERS

Widowed Spouse

I am currently one of the organizers, founders, and co-facilitators of our Parkinson's support group.

My husband had Parkinson's disease (PD) for almost 20 years. He was diagnosed at age 55 and died at age 74. He was diagnosed in 1992 and died on September 1, 2011.

He told me he was experiencing weakness on his left side. I urged him to go to a doctor because his father had died at a young age of heart disease. His internist recommended he go for several tests. The tests ruled out heart disease, so he thought he should see a neurologist in case he possibly had a pinched nerve. The general neurologist observed he was holding his left arm at an odd angle. It was hanging and not swinging naturally by his side, and he walked kind of shuffling at a rather slow gait. The neurologist suspected that he might have Parkinson's and put him on medication to see if that would help. If it did help, he said, it would indicate he had Parkinson's. There was no other way to test for it.

When he told me, he said, "I have Parkinson's disease." It came out of the blue. I was really kind of not knowing how to react. Neither one of us knew much about the disease. He said, "You could have told me I was pregnant and I wouldn't have been more surprised."

When I think back, it was confusion that made me decide, more so than him, to find out as much as I could about the disease. He could not have cared less at that point. I looked for different resources at the library, but most of the information was difficult to wade through because of the medical terminology. His doctor was not too helpful telling us what we might expect along the way. I learned he was lacking dopamine, a chemical that controls movement. We had no past history or family history of PD.

My husband was functioning real well, but eventually he did tell his boss about the diagnosis. His boss assured him they would be behind him and help him handle things if the disease progressed.

His health got put on the back burner, but with added Parkinson's medication, I began to notice behavioral changes, such that he was becoming highly egotistical. He was very creative, but he became very outgoing and boisterous about his accomplishments. He wanted the attention. That was very much unlike him. Gambling came into the picture. He couldn't' stay out of the casinos. That was very unlike him. Also, he became very highly sexual. He had all three of those compulsive behaviors. I became alarmed about this, and we talked to the neurologist. I thought there was a connection to one of the medications. Now, they're very aware of it and don't use that medication any more, but at that time, the doctor dismissed it as a midlife crisis. I couldn't accept that. I knew it was the medication, but I had to do a lot of research to find the connection. Way down on the list of possible side effects of agonists was "compulsive behavior."

One thing led to another. I thought I was going crazy.

Meanwhile, my husband loved to write and was writing part-time. He decided to write full-time, and also maintain his job, but on a part-time basis. After only a month, he told me he had been let go. He lost his job supposedly because of sexual harassment. Someone complained because he was talking to other women about OUR sexual relationship. The company fired him after an exemplary 30 year career in advertising and marketing. He had received many awards for developing creative and innovative advertising campaigns. They didn't have much of a case against him. It seemed a way for the company to get out of paying disability. It put a lot of stress on our relationship and our finances, too. I was retiring as a part-time teacher. We didn't even qualify for Social Security yet.

So, we started a little publishing company. We put money from our savings into it. Looking back, it helped our relationship for me to handle the business end, and we travelled together to promote the books we published.

After he was fired, we decided to bring a suit against the company for improper dismissal. It is a small company. We had a lawyer. We decided to settle out of court for an amount equal to two years salary. One-third went to the lawyer, one-third to taxes. But, the hardest part was losing the friendships we had made throughout the years with the company. My husband was very angry. So was I, about the whole thing. He didn't want to stay in the same area as the company, even though we'd been there about ten years. He wanted to move back closer to family.

When we moved back 15 years ago, we needed to find a new neurologist. We noticed there was a seminar being given by the Michigan Parkinson Foundation. We asked people at the seminar who they went to for a doctor. A couple of movement disorder specialists' names were given us. Within five minutes of seeing our new neurologist and telling him about my husband's behavioral problems, the doctor said, "It's the medication." I asked him specifically why the highly regarded neurologist we had been seeing couldn't make the connection between the behavior and the medication. He said he probably didn't have enough Parkinson's patients to know.

It was a huge relief to know that it was the medication causing his behavior. All along, I knew something wasn't right, and it was a relief to find a doctor who was knowledgeable about the disease.

My husband wasn't able to control his behavior when he was on the medication. He still required additional medication as a supplement, but, in his case, additional medication would always trigger the compulsive behaviors. He wasn't able to grasp that his behavior was so out of control and inappropriate. He thought that his behavior was OK.

We went to a priest we knew, and he referred us to a social worker. Together, we went to counseling with a social worker that was excellent.

Other symptoms he suffered were physical, such as rigidity in his leg and arm at first, and eventually in both legs and arms. Our neurologist recommended we look into Deep Brain Stimulation (DBS) surgery to help reduce the amount of meds he'd have to take. DBS was still in clinical trials at that time. After talking with my husband, the neurosurgeon who was doing the DBS trials determined he would be a good candidate for the surgery. This was in 2000. The doctor let him into the trials – which were coming to an end. Within two months, the FDA approved the surgery. He couldn't wait. He would have gone the next day. I was the one saying, "Hey, this is brain surgery."

After the surgery, and after making adjustments to the wired settings, he was able to lower the amount of meds he used, and he didn't need any agonist. He seemed to do pretty well. He didn't have as much rigidity and he had more movement. In my opinion, I think DBS extended his quality of life by five or more years. He could still play golf and write, and we travelled a little. The thing he liked to do most of all was play the piano.

After his DBS surgery, he wrote a book chronicling his journey with PD and his DBS surgical experience. We traveled to PD support groups throughout the state to speak about his book and the relatively new surgical procedure. We saw the need for a support group in our area and, with the help of two other interested people, we organized a group. That was eight years ago.

Even though he was stabilized by DBS and on just one medication, the disease still progressed, though slowly.

Between 2001 and 2011, additional things came into the picture like shuffling, and balance problems. He fell a lot. His cognition deteriorated. He had mild hallucinations due to drugs he needed for his rigidity so that he could keep moving. He had mild dyskinesia. Then he really went downhill – with his falling. He was 6'1" and weighed 180 pounds. Trying to lift him or help him get up when he fell was impossible.

This is where I tell caregivers that anger is one of the steps of grief you go through. "Why Me?" you ask. It's a long, long journey to acceptance. You're losing part of them along the way, and you're also trying to keep yourself together. I developed a part of the house that was just mine – where I could read or use the computer.

His swallowing became a problem. He'd cough after eating. He started losing his speech. It was difficult to understand him. His voice was slurry and like a mumble. Drooling was a problem. He wore a beard to camouflage it somewhat. Sometimes it would be really bad and sometimes not. Physically, he had the masked face ten years into it, about 1998, and apathy set in. He didn't have feelings for things.

I was his social director. I tried to keep something to shoot for every day. He'd ask, "What do we have on the calendar today?" We did things like go to the library. We went out every day for lunch. We made many trips to a Metro park. We called it, "going up north." We'd take a lunch, take a radio, and listen to music. He looked forward to it.

As he progressed, he lost his ability to concentrate. He could no longer play games or stay with a task. I'd set up a project for him, and by the time I laid it out, he'd forget how to do it.

Dementia came on slowly. He'd get days mixed up. He was getting so he'd forget where the bathroom was in our condo we'd lived in for six years. He'd put his clothes on backwards. Humor is a big thing – laughing at things that happen.

What really took him down was when he got a urinary tract infection early in 2011. About three months after the infection cleared up, it came back. He was not able to eliminate. It took a week to get in to see the urologist. He started running a temperature, he couldn't walk, and he was disoriented. EMS took us to emergency. They drained off 1800 CC's of urine that he'd been retaining in his system. He was admitted into the hospital for this infection and was put on antibiotics. He was in the hospital eating pureed food because of difficulty swallowing. The infection was not clearing up and he was getting weaker and weaker. After about four days, he was put on a Foley catheter. They advised that he should go to a rehab facility to get stronger. He was doing OK there, but he wasn't gaining his strength back. Then they noticed the infection was back again. They put him on a stronger antibiotic. His strength was zapping away. A sore on his bottom was becoming quite infected. He had to go back into the hospital to have that looked at. He was too weak for surgery, so they tried to clear it up with antibiotics. They put him back in the rehab nursing center. To stay on Medicare, you have to show improvement, but he wasn't, so they moved him into skilled nursing – the nursing home part of the facility. They had to use a lift to put him into a chair because he was too weak to stand without assistance.

I used to tool him around in his wheel chair. They had ice cream every afternoon. Our social worker was a daughter of good friends of ours. Her dad has PD, too. She really oversaw things for us, and gave us knowledgeable information. It was like God had a personal hand on us.

I knew I'd never be able to bring him home the way he was. I wouldn't be able to get him up if he fell.

He went into the hospital with the UTI in late June. He died September 1st. The infection was still raging and he was getting weaker and weaker. His extremities were always cold, and his blood flow was not good.

Because of the ravages of the infection, his whole system was deteriorating. His neurologist said it was very common for PD patients to have urinary tract infections. By this time, my husband couldn't do anything. He couldn't even communicate well. That afternoon we were watching a ball game. I always stayed for supper and brushed his teeth for him. I thought he was dozing in his chair. His head had dropped lower on his chest than usual. I got no response when I tried to shake him. The nurse came in and said, "I think he's gone." He was peaceful. He was 74. I had been losing him little by little by little for the last two years. It was such a shock, but it was a relief that he wouldn't have to deal with this anymore.

I'd already done a lot of grieving along the way.

Those months in the nursing/rehab center were the best months we had together. I didn't have the stress of taking care of him 24 hours. I could sit with him in the beautiful garden. Those last days together, we talked and reminisced about the fun we'd had, and the accordion he'd played at Polish weddings when we were young. We have three sons, two granddaughters and a grandson whom he loved dearly. It was a consoling time. I think more of those good times than all the previous bad times.

The biggest challenge as a caregiver was trying to have patience on a daily basis. There were times when it was thin, and, yes, I did yell and get nasty occasionally. At the end of the day I would always give him a big kiss, and apologize, and say, "I'm just so mad at this disease." He said, "I understand. I am, too."

My spiritual life was greatly enhanced by this experience. I had to have someone I could turn to each morning and pray, "Guide me today to do the best I can." My faith has become so much stronger. I use the *Serenity Prayer*, "Grant me the serenity to accept the things I cannot change, the courage to change the things I can, and the wisdom to know the difference."

I particularly remember one day nearing our 50th anniversary. I had to drop him off at the library. When I came to get him, I searched inside for him but couldn't find him. His balance was getting poor. He didn't have his cell phone. He used somebody's phone to call me to say, "I'm downtown. Come pick me up." I was boiling angry. I was so worried. When I picked him up, there he was with a huge bouquet of flowers. He'd walked to a florist, limited as he was. How can you be mad at that? There were so many times I'd leave him in the car for ten minutes, he'd take off, try to come and look for me, go inside a store, fall, and they would have to call EMS to pick him up.

Advice to caretakers:

- Have someone that will just listen to you, someone to talk to without them trying to fix it or help you.

- Take it day by day – hour by hour.

- Have something you can do for yourself every day, even if you don't go outside the house. Usually for me it was 9 p.m. when he'd go to bed. On Friday night, after I got him tucked in, I'd have what I called "Party Night," with wine, cheese, and my favorite book.

- Humor is important. To get him to walk, I'd have to play drill sergeant, "left, right, left, right."

If people aren't going through the same experience, they won't really understand. That's why caregiver's support groups are great. There we can talk about immediate concerns and feel like, "These people really do know what I'm talking about."

Through my involvement with PD, I realize how important education is. "Knowledge is Power," and being a former educator, it sort of fit that I would want to gain knowledge about the disease and want to pass it along to help others on their journey.

MAKE THE MOST OF MOMENTS YOU HAVE

Widowed Spouse

They noticed at work that he was dragging his one foot. It was 1980. He was diagnosed with Parkinson's disease (PD) at age 50. It was 22 years ago that he died. He would have turned 64 one month later.

I noticed a tremor in his hand. We were having a cocktail one night and his hand shook while he was holding his glass. He had been working hard in the yard all day, and he said, "Oh, this tremor is just a little muscle fatigue from all the yard work I've been doing." So, we just chalked it up to that.

He was always very athletic and coordinated. We were cross country skiing with friends and his left leg wanted to go out, like he couldn't track. His friends said, "Maybe you need to get some new skis or new bindings."

We didn't do anything about it for probably almost another year.

Then he called me from work one day. He said he was due for his physical and he was going in because his co-workers noticed that when he walked, his left leg seemed to drag. Later he called me and said, "What do you know about Parkinson's disease?"

I said, "Parkinson's?" I thought of the PD patients I helped during my nurse's training. I just remembered they were all older, shuffling, and drooling, with tremors in their hands. I just couldn't imagine a 50 year old healthy man coming down with Parkinson's. I was shocked. Number 1, he wasn't old, number 2, I had no idea about "young onset" Parkinson's. I felt I needed to get to know more about the illness. He didn't know anything either. He was shocked, and I guess frightened, too. But, he was still functioning.

Originally, it didn't affect our lifestyle. He continued to fly his airplane. The last time we were up in the airplane, I recognized that we were coming in too fast for the landing. He was "frozen," and I jolted him to come out of it. I had to help him land. Then he realized that maybe it wasn't that safe for him to fly anymore. That was about four years after his diagnosis.

He was diagnosed in 1980. He retired in 1982 on medical retirement. We moved to Tennessee in 1984 to a complex where a lot of automotive people had retired to. We thought he could stay more active because of the activities there, and milder winters. We lived there for over five years, but after four years the kids could see changes happening to him. I was the sole caregiver there, and they wanted us to come back so they could be more involved in their dad's life and be a help to me.

He had always been a very expressive person with a strong personality. He was 6'2." His appearance changed. He shuffled. He had the flat affect of the face. He had the Parkinson's stare and lack of facial expression. He was fine when the meds were working. The meds helped him feel good and be free of his rigidity. But, sometimes, he would get so loose he would have big movements and facial grimacing.

It was strange, because his reaction to the meds were very different. He was either "on" or "off." When he felt good, he would just want to take off. Otherwise, he would be so rigid that he could hardly make a step forward. Then the meds would kick in, and I could predict that within five minutes, he would be able to manage the steps and take off. Of course, it would fade just as fast. That's when he would have problems falling. In other words, he was so sensitive to the meds that it was hard to keep him on an even plane.

I think the hardest part to accept was the drastic change in our lifestyle. We had always been so social and active. Suddenly we became isolated because of his tremors and the change in his personality, which was a side effect of the meds. He was such a proud man and became embarrassed with his speech pattern and his inability to express himself. He would try, but he couldn't get his thoughts out. One day he said, "Give me a pencil and let me write it." But, he started out writing and it became a straight line, so he couldn't write either. It was more toward the end that he had the problem of not really being able to communicate. He had a lot of anger and frustration.

The caregiver's life definitely changes, too. I was isolated because I felt I couldn't leave him alone. I eventually called the hospital for home care. I had someone come out a couple times a week for four hours each to bathe him and shower him and stay so I could go shopping or pull myself together. I might go and just sit and look at a book in the library.

I got a lot of support from my children. I did have two occasions when I got away. One was through a "Well Spouse" organization – a group of caregivers. There, I met a lot of people who were also caregivers of Parkinson's patients. It was a break for me, and I knew he was well taken care of by the children. He always thought I was fleeing from him and running away, though. That upset him.

Anything different or unusual for him increased his anxiety level. I think it was hard for him to relinquish things to me, but he loved travelling, so he had to turn over certain things, such as driving our motor home. We kept that up until the end.

I think there are many different levels of Parkinson's. It's easy to think they could do more for themselves, because the tasks seem so simple to us. If the Parkinson's patient is a man who has always had an image of being in control, and being needed, I think it can be a problem when the role is reversed. You want to encourage them to be as independent as possible, but it's easier to do for them, because they have such a difficult time, and because they're so slow. Taking over for them, however, affects their pride and cuts down on their ability to do for themselves.

Everything slows down with PD, including the digestive process, the respiratory process, and the circulation. Extremities become colder. Swallowing was difficult, as was the digestion of food. I had to be a lot more careful with his diet. And, the evacuation process – the bowels – can become impacted.

I was a Registered Nurse, and most of my career was spent in public health. I was also a medical/surgical nurse. I eventually had to retire because of his illness. At the time, what I did was very much curtailed because of caring for him.

Our circle of friends became smaller. He could no longer play bridge. He would be his old self one minute, and all of a sudden, he'd be rigid and couldn't communicate, and he'd go lay down. Our good times were measured in minutes instead of hours. You could sense our friends didn't know how to deal with it. He knew he was different, too, and he kind of withdrew. He would tire easily. He was so different than he had been before the PD. I attributed his psychological problems to the side effects of the meds. He would become combative, or run away. I attribute the depression to the disease.

I would advise caregivers to become knowledgeable about the disease. So often, others don't have the foggiest idea of what PD is, other than what they can visually see. Find out how meds affect the Parkinson's patient. Each person reacts differently.

I would also advise the caregiver to take a break from the constant togetherness.

We may like to think we can handle anything, and that we can deal with what life has dealt us, but I tried to take advantage of the help that was available. The support groups are a place you can get suggestions from people going through the same thing as you are.

Caregivers and patients need to have separate support groups so each has a chance to express feelings that they wouldn't otherwise express.

Don't shut out your family, thinking you're protecting them. The kids were very concerned about their dad, and they did not understand his illness. They were scared and wondered if the same thing might happen to me, so they sometimes put on blinders. Get more help from them if you can, even though you hate to call on them because they're raising their own families and dealing with their jobs.

It's hard to see a loved one deteriorate. The final goodbyes are kind of a mixed blessing. You know they're no longer suffering, but you miss them.

In hindsight, I can't help but have some guilt feelings, wondering if I could have done more. Could I have taken him to a different doctor? Should I have done this or that?

He died at home. The last neurologist said there was nothing more that could be done. The meds were no longer effective. They were doing more harm than good. He was rapidly losing weight. We took him off the meds. He would become very rigid. I put him in hospice care. The doctor for hospice put him on morphine every four hours, until the end. I had mixed feelings as I was the one administering this drug to my husband, knowing it was speeding up the end of his life. I was just trying to keep him comfortable.

We met at age 14. We lived a block from one another. Our parents were friends.

GIVING BACK IN MEMORY OF LOVED ONES

Daughter of Parkinson's Patient (deceased)

When my father passed away, I moved my mother from her home into an apartment condo in the same area. Even though I knew I would be her caregiver and lived a good distance away, I thought it best she stay near her friends.

As she aged, I felt something was really wrong. She started shuffling her feet, staring out the window, and she became rather paranoid about everything. Her face became stoic. At that point, I felt I needed to have questions answered. Had she suffered a stroke? What was wrong with her? I took her to a neurologist and his conclusion was that she had Parkinson's disease (PD). It was 1991 and she was 78 years old. The doctor prescribed levodopa. I knew nothing about PD and didn't know where to turn for help. I only had the little information the doctor gave us about the possible progression of the disease.

One morning my mother woke up and proceeded to get out of bed. She sat in her bedside chair. From that point on, she was totally "frozen" for almost ten hours. She was finally able to take her bedside lamp and bang it against the apartment wall until someone heard her. The police were called, and they had to break into her apartment to help her. They called me to inform me. At that point, I knew it was not safe for her to live alone.

Her life was not easy from then on. We hired a full time live-in caregiver for her, and I continued to commute daily to oversee her life. The paranoia she suffered was awful. She also lost her appetite, and she had constant urinary tract infections.

She ended up in a nursing home with a permanent catheter. She could no longer swallow and was put into hospice care. She passed away on her birthday in 1996 at the age of 83.

My father-in-law was also diagnosed with PD by his eye doctor in 1972. He didn't have tremors, but he shuffled and had the masked stare. He insisted on living alone. He passed after falling and hitting his head on the bathroom sink. It was 1974. He was 86.

My advice to caregivers is, try to find a local Parkinson's support group and a caregiver's support group, and learn about ways to take care of your loved one. Find out about doctors who specialize in movement disorders. I joined the Parkinson's support group to support the facilitator and her husband and also to give back through fund raising in memory of my mother and father-in-law. I have made many new acquaintances, learned a lot about the disease, and gained an understanding of what I did not know when my mother and father-in-law were diagnosed.

ACKNOWLEDGEMENTS

Nat Upton: My brother, for being on call all hours of the day and night, for editing and consulting, and for helping solve computer problems.

Kristi Henry: For helping proofread, and spending hours with me on the computer formatting for publishing.

Carl Virgilio: For designing and laying out cover.

Harriett Marenas: For being a creative stimulus always, and being an encouraging and interested friend. She suggested I write this book, and she suggested I include a poem, which I did.

Nancy Knitter: For being my "go to" person; for finding pertinent reference information, but most of all, for being our tireless support group leader.

Janet Lang: For always being available and willing to read for clarification, grammar and punctuation.

Alan Thebert: For being willing to help proofread.

Lori Frye: For being a supportive friend.

MOST OF ALL, MY HEROES: The Parkinson's patients and their spouses and loved ones, for "being the book," by sharing so honestly and openly in our intimate conversations.

PARKINSON'S DISEASE RESOURCES

American Parkinson Disease Association
www.apdaparkinson.org
(800) 223-2732

Caregiver.com
(800) 829-2734

Caregiver Action Network (CAN)
www.caregiveraction.org
(202) 772-5050

DaTscan™
www.datscan.com

Davis Phinney Foundation
www.davisphinneyfoundation.org
(866) 358-0285

Lewy Body Dementia Association, Inc.
www.lbda.org
(800) 539-9767

LSVT Global, Inc.
www.lsvtglobal.com
(888) 438-5788

The Michael J. Fox Foundation
www.michaeljfox.org
(800) 708-7644

Michigan Parkinson Foundation
www.parkinsonsmi.org
(800) 852-9781

The Movement Disorder Society
www.movementdisorders.org
(414) 276-2145

Muhammed Ali Parkinson Center
www.thebarrow.org
(800) 227-7691

National Caregiving Foundation
www.caregivingfoundation.org
(800) 930-1357

National Parkinson Foundation
www.parkinson.org
(800) 327-4545

Northwest Parkinson's Foundation
www.nwpf.org
(877) 980-7500

Parkinson's Action Network (PAN)
www.parkinsonsaction.org
(800) 850-4726

Parkinson's Disease Foundation
www.pdf.org
(800) 457-6676

Parkinson Society Canada
www.parkinson.ca
(416) 227-9700
(800) 565-3000

GLOSSARY

Bradykinesia
One of the cardinal clinical features of Parkinson's disease, the slowing down and loss of spontaneous and voluntary movement. From the Greek *brady*, slow, and *kinesia*, movement.

DaTscan™
DaTscan is an imaging drug that will be injected into the bloodstream to help your doctor assess a chemical in your brain called dopamine. A special device, called a gamma camera, will take pictures of your brain. These pictures and/or a report will be sent to your doctor, who can discuss the test results with you.

The DaTscan is the only FDA-approved imaging drug available that provides an image your doctor can view to help determine – in combination with an assessment of symptoms and possibly other tests – if you may be suffering from Parkinsonian syndromes or another condition with similar symptoms called essential tremor.

Deep brain stimulation
Deep brain stimulation (DBS) is a surgical procedure that uses a surgically implanted, battery-operated medical device called a neurostimulator – similar to a heart pacemaker and approximately the size of a stopwatch – to deliver electrical stimulation to targeted areas in the brain that control movement, blocking the abnormal nerve signals that cause tremor and PD symptoms. At present, the procedure is used primarily for patients whose symptoms cannot be satisfactorily controlled with medication.

Dopamine
A neurotransmitter chemical produced in the brain that helps control movement, balance, and walking. Lack of dopamine is the primary cause of Parkinson's motor symptoms.

Dopamine agonist
A class of drugs commonly prescribed for Parkinson's disease that bind to dopamine receptors and mimic dopamine's actions in the brain. Dopamine agonists stimulate dopamine receptors and produce dopamine-like effects.

Dyskinesia
Involuntary, uncontrollable, and often excessive movements that are a common side effect of levodopa treatment for Parkinson's disease. These movements can be lurching, dance-like or jerky, and are distinct from the rhythmic tremor commonly associated with Parkinson's disease.

Facial masking
A symptom experienced by some people with Parkinson's, in which the face is immobile with reduced blinking. Also referred to as hypomimia.

Festination
An involuntary quickening of steps and shuffling after starting to walk. Festination is a common feature of Parkinson's disease.

Freezing
Abrupt and temporary inability of Parkinson's patients to move that frequently occurs when beginning to walk or at a boundary such as a door or when exiting a car.

Hoehn and Yahr Scale
1 - Symptoms on only one side of the body.
2 - Symptoms on both sides of the body and no difficulty walking.
3 - Symptoms on both sides of the body and minimal difficulty walking.
4 - Symptoms on both sides of the body and moderate difficulty walking.
5 - Symptoms on both sides of the body and unable to walk.

InterStim therapy
A proven neuromodulator therapy that targets the communication problem between the brain and the nerves that control the bladder. (Medtronics)

Levodopa
Also called L-dopa, the most commonly administered drug to treat Parkinson's symptoms. Levodopa helps restore levels of dopamine, a chemical messenger in the brain responsible for smooth, coordinated movement and other motor and cognitive functions.

Lewy Bodies
Abnormal protein clumps that accumulate in dead or dying dopamine-producing cells of the substantia nigra in Parkinson's disease. At autopsy, the presence of Lewy bodies is used to confirm a Parkinson's diagnosis.

LSVT® BIG
An intensive physical and occupational therapy exercise program for people with Parkinson Disease and other neurological conditions. Treatments target the production of larger amplitude whole body functional movements while retraining the sensory awareness of the effort required for normal movement.

LSVT® LOUD.
An effective speech treatment for individuals with Parkinson disease (PD) and other neurological conditions. LSVT® LOUD, named for Mrs. Lee Silverman (Lee Silverman Voice Treatment – LSVT®) was developed in 1987 and has been scientifically studied for nearly 20 years with funding support from the National Institute for Deafness and other Communication Disorders (NIDCD) of the National Institutes of Health. LSVT® LOUD improves vocal loudness by stimulating the muscles of the voice box (larynx) and speech mechanism through a systematic hierarchy of exercises.

MRSA
MRSA is a "staph" germ that does not get better with the first-line antibiotics that usually cure staph infections. Most staph germs are spread by skin-to-skin contact (touching). A doctor, nurse, other health care provider, or visitors may have staph germs on their body that can spread to a patient.

Neupro skin patch (rotigotine)
Has some of the same effects as a chemical called dopamine. Low levels of dopamine in the brain are associated with Parkinson's disease. They are used to treat symptoms of Parkinson's disease, such as stiffness, tremors, muscle spasms, and poor muscle control. Neupro is also used to treat restless legs syndrome (RLS).

On – Off Phenomenon
Sudden loss of activity of levodopa lasting minutes to hours after a brief period of effectiveness. The term also sometimes refers to a cyclical response to medication where the patient can function adequately at times but is too stiff and immobile to function at other times

Parkinson's disease

Parkinson's disease is a chronic, degenerative neurological disorder that affects one in 100 people over age 60. While the average age at onset is 60, people have been diagnosed as young as 18. There is no objective test, or biomarker, for Parkinson's disease, so the rate of misdiagnosis can be relatively high, especially when the diagnosis is made by a non-specialist. Estimates of the number of people living with the disease therefore vary, but recent research indicates that at least one million people in the United States, and more than five million worldwide, have Parkinson's disease.

Parkinsonism

Generic term referring to slowness and mobility problems that result from or look like Parkinson's disease. Several conditions that are not actually Parkinson's disease, including multiple system atrophy and progressive supranuclear palsy, as well as a number of medications, can result in parkinsonism and a misdiagnosis of Parkinson's disease.

Postural instability

Uncontrollable problems with standing or walking, or impaired balance and coordination, which are symptoms of Parkinson's disease for some patients and do not respond to dopamine replacement therapy.

Restless leg syndrome

An urge or desire to move their legs, usually accompanied by unpleasant or disagreeable sensations such as numbness, tingling, crawling, itching, aching, burning, cramping, or pain.

Sinemet

The brand name of the most commonly prescribed version of the drug levodopa, consisting of a combination of levodopa and carbidopa.

Sundowning
The term "sundowning" refers to a state of confusion at the end of the day and into the night. Sundowning isn't a disease, but a symptom that often occurs in people with dementia, such as Alzheimer's disease. The cause isn't known.

Tremor
Involuntary, uncontrollable, rhythmic movements (fast or slow) that may affect the hands, head, voice or other body parts. Resting tremor is one of the cardinal clinical features of Parkinson's disease.

Uveitis
An inflammation of the middle layer of the eye (the uvea), but in common usage, it refers to all inflammatory processes inside the eye.
(Cleveland Clinic)

Wearing off
A loss of effectiveness of Parkinson's medications between doses. If the effectiveness of a medication does not last until the next dose is due, it "wears off."

Definitions were obtained from various sources, including The Michael J. Fox Foundation, the Mayo Clinic, Medtronic, the Cleveland Clinic, LSVT Global, GE Healthcare, and the National Institute of Health.

Medical Disclaimer

This book should not be used as a substitute for professional medical advice. Parkinson's disease, and its symptoms, may vary with each individual. A neurologist specializing in Parkinson's disease and movement disorders should be consulted in matters related to your health, particularly with respect to any symptoms that may require diagnosis or medical attention.

ORDER INFORMATION

To order *Behind the Mask of Parkinson's Disease*,
please contact us at:

Behind the Mask
P.O. Box 82365
Rochester, MI 48308

Or email: ParkinsonsBook@comcast.net

Books are also available online through
www.createspace.com
www.amazon.com

Checks, payable to *Behind the Mask*, and credit card
orders will be accepted.

ABOUT THE AUTHOR

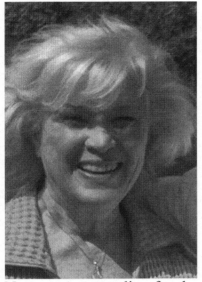

Lavonne Upton was diagnosed with Parkinson's disease in August of 2011. Her knowledge of this degenerative disease preceded her diagnosis, however, having two brothers with Parkinson's, one of whom died from complications of the disease.

Never content settling for the status quo, she has taken on new challenges with verve and energy to become a multi-faceted, multi-talented woman who enjoys writing.

Lavonne Upton is an involved mother of two and grandmother of five. In both her personal and professional lives, she has built on her experiences to explore new opportunities.

As a writer, she has written a monthly column for several community journals and worked as a free-lance photo-journalist for a daily newspaper. She is a contributing author to *Heart of a Mother* and *Heart of the Holidays* in the Heart Book Series. She also published *What Would* THIS *Granny Do,* under the pen name of emma lavonne, which is currently available through amazon.com, and createspace.com.

52950056R00151

Made in the USA
Lexington, KY
16 June 2016